HEALED BY HIS HAND:
BODY, MIND, AND SPIRIT

KARSEN DELGADO, FNP - C

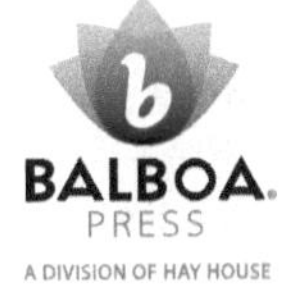

BALBOA
PRESS
A DIVISION OF HAY HOUSE

Scripture taken from the New King James Version. Copyright © 1979, 1980, 1982 by Thomas Nelson, Inc. Used by permission. All rights reserved.

Balboa Press books may be ordered through booksellers or by contacting:

Balboa Press
A Division of Hay House
1663 Liberty Drive
Bloomington, IN 47403
www.balboapress.com
1 (877) 407-4847

Because of the dynamic nature of the Internet, any web addresses or links contained in this book may have changed since publication and may no longer be valid. The views expressed in this work are solely those of the author and do not necessarily reflect the views of the publisher, and the publisher hereby disclaims any responsibility for them.

The author of this book does not dispense medical advice or prescribe the use of any technique as a form of treatment for physical, emotional, or medical problems without the advice of a physician, either directly or indirectly. The intent of the author is only to offer information of a general nature to help you in your quest for emotional and spiritual well-being. In the event you use any of the information in this book for yourself, which is your constitutional right, the author and the publisher assume no responsibility for your actions.

Any people depicted in stock imagery provided by Getty Images are models, and such images are being used for illustrative purposes only. Certain stock imagery © Getty Images.

Print information available on the last page.

ISBN: 978-1-9822-0508-9 (sc)
ISBN: 978-1-9822-0507-2 (hc)
ISBN: 978-1-9822-0509-6 (e)

Library of Congress Control Number: 2018906239

Balboa Press rev. date: 06/11/2018

Author's Note

This book is dedicated to my Savior Jesus Christ, Heavenly Mother, and Heavenly Father. Thank you for your divine love. And to my terrenal parents- Thank you for giving me this life, love and guidance along the way. To my spouse- thank you for being my eternal companion, now and forever.

Contents

Introduction

This book is designed to educate the reader on how God has revealed to me His way of healing. Christ is the True Healer and He uses His power to help others turn to Him, change their lives and heal on a deep physical, spiritual and emotional level. We have, over the ages, focused more on the physical aspects of healing, as opposed to the emotional and spiritual. We recognize the connection, but have not yet accessed the greater power that lies within us to heal, as we focus more on the spiritual and emotional components He has given to us.

It is my hope and prayer that as you study these words, the Spirit will enlighten your mind, fill you with faith, and ignite your soul as you pursue the path to true healing. It is by design that these concepts were brought about in our day so that you can be made whole *now*. I encourage you to ask for an open mind and heart so that this information can bring remembrance of things previously learned to your awareness. As you allow the Holy Spirit into your life and align to God's truth in all things, you will be filled with light and all darkness will dissipate, removing illness and pain, and restoring you to full health.

Several people have questioned why there is so much suffering in the world, and why there are those who have prolonged suffering. Many feel that it's simply God's will that they have to learn through their trial of experience. Indeed, we are required to learn and experience a variety of things that promote growth and understanding. However, it has been made known to me that many times the trial of sickness is prolonged when the individual could have already been made whole. This delay in a full restoration of health has occurred because of the limited understanding of men in science and health, and the subsequent production of therapies that are designed to manage symptoms instead of treating the true etiology. All of these factors dampen faith and weaken our resolve to change things that may be contributing, or even causing our symptoms.

When we take a medication, we are sending the message to our body that the underlying condition needs to be managed, but not healed. We also limit our faith by depending on the knowledge of man instead of the wisdom and knowledge of God. We can pray for discernment to acknowledge the truth from the error and align ourselves directly to God's laws of healing. We can indeed reject the "wiles of the adversary" which include false belief systems about health, limited and flawed testing capabilities, and fear inducing procedures or recommendations. The more we align and adhere to the truth in all things- the more we will be empowered to heal through Christ's power.

It takes *work* to develop the faith necessary to be fully restored to health, and therefore medications *can* support the individual where they are at on the continuum of faith and development. Also, specific dietary changes and supplements can be incorporated as indicated by the Spirit that can fill us with more light, hope and faith. In Scripture, the Savior says, *"And again, it shall come to pass that he that hath FAITH in me to be healed, and is **not** appointed unto death, shall be healed."* Doctrine and Covenants 42:48.

Do you believe it? Do you believe that you can truly heal from any and all emotional, spiritual and physical distress through the power of God? I **know** you can. If the belief has not come to fruition yet, you can ask that *all* genes of faith in God, faith in self, faith to be healed, and faith to heal be turned on. There are many genes of faith and this is the starting point.

If one is appointed unto death, then the process of healing will not occur. It is important to ask the Lord if He desires you to be healed at this time so you may know that it is possible. You may be told "not yet," and it may be because there are still certain things for you to learn through the experience. If that is your answer, then there are specific spiritual gifts and abilities you can ask for to help you better manage the experience such as the gift of patience, persistence and long suffering. But, if you feel that the trial of health should be over and He affirms it to be so, know that you can silence beliefs that contributed to the illness to begin with, fortify the immune system to finish destroying the pathogens related to your problem, and turn on genes of faith, light, hope and love which will blot out the darkness of disease.

I cannot underscore the importance of the heart and mind in this process. Faith promoting meditations and pondering of scripture were essential to my ability to heal. Removing the stressors and demands of time, and allowing things to be simplified and slowed were important as well. You may feel prompted to let go of physical activity and exercise to dedicate your energies to healing physically. You may have already needed to give up physical activity- yet this is a great opportunity to exercise the power of the *mind*.

The mind is the gateway to our soul, and what we allow ourselves to think on, ponder, and meditate about channels those emotions into our very sinews. Literally, our emotions and thoughts affect gene expression of the spiritual DNA! Similarly, those encoded spiritual proteins affect the expression of the physical DNA. Thus, negativity in the forms of fear, anger, frustration, regret, envy, greed, and disbelief (and more) will pull us down and prevent us from fully healing. Filling the mind with faith, hope, charity, kindness, patience, gratitude, and belief (and more) will raise us up to the level of light needed for true healing to occur.

In regards to my background and experience, I have always had a love of learning. From a very young age, I was driven and dedicated to the study of creations, science, and the earth. I felt very drawn to biology, chemistry, anatomy and physiology, and felt wonder and awe as I delved deeper into the underlying meaning of God's creations.

A deep reverence came over me as I pondered His meaning of these things, and the symbolism associated with the smallest of creations, down to the atom. Throughout my life, He has guided me and directed me to the truth, **His** truth of the mysteries of the world, by granting me the gift of discernment.

I felt prompted to pursue nursing as a career and loved to nurture and help His children in their afflictions. It gave me great joy and a greater understanding of God's love for each of us. After obtaining my registered nurse associate degree, I served an LDS mission in Ecuador and was called to minister to the missionaries serving in that capacity, providing recommendations of what they could do to improve their physical and emotional health. I saw parallels between physical health and spiritual well being during this time, but nothing like what has been unfolding before me at present.

After my mission, I met my wonderful husband and continued to pursue my education. I obtained my Bachelor's degree in Nursing at Weber State University, followed by my Master's degree at Brigham Young University. I studied for my boards and successfully passed them in October of 2008. I was officially a Family Nurse Practitioner, and thrilled to have been granted this opportunity in higher learning and a new application of skills. During this time we hoped for a family, but I was unable to conceive. It was a trial for me, but as I was immersed in study and reflection, I trusted the Lord's timetable.

Shortly after graduation from Brigham Young University, I found out I was pregnant. It was a wonderful experience and I loved being part of creation— feeling the baby move, learning about his personality even prior to his birth, and so much more. All these emotions and feelings of becoming a new mother filled me with joy and gratitude. The delivery did not go as planned at all. I was faced with a caesarean section after 26 hours of labor and failure to progress. The recovery was still fairly quick despite the pain of the incision, and I was so grateful to have my beautiful baby boy. However, shortly thereafter, something changed. I began to have insomnia and agitation, which then became severe anxiety and panic.

I couldn't eat and I was always on edge. It was if adrenaline was coursing through my veins 24 hours a day.

During this debilitating time, I experienced the worst emotional, physical and spiritual turmoil of my life. It was definitely a refiner's fire and I learned to rely on the Lord as I never had before. I relied on the testimony of others, and clung to the hope that I would be well again, and that this state of anxiety would not be the rest of my life. Time slowed down, I learned to take one day at a time, sometimes one minute at a time. I strived so hard to seek out positivity, and tried with fervor to change the negative spiraling thoughts into light towards Christ and His suffering. I focused on serving others and looking upward and outward, despite my severe sleep deprivation and malnutrition. Through service to others, I was filled with Christ's love, and eventually things settled back down to normalcy.

This experience was so extreme that I sought out help from medical professionals. At the time, I only knew one way to treat illness and emotional distress— through medications. Thus I started on medication and it helped mitigate the symptoms of my mood disorder, but did not heal me from it. I remember distinctly thinking I would get off of it when I was done having children, like it would be a crutch and a support for me, but not the end-all to my healing.

I worked in a Family practice/Community Health Center during these years and I LOVED it!! During this time, I was able to dedicate myself to further study and investigation for patients who had limited resources and funds. As providers in this location, we were called upon to serve many roles: the endocrinologist, the gastroenterologist, the neurologist, and dermatologist. Our patients could not afford to go to specialists, and I appreciated the opportunity to grow. However, I only sought out information scientifically according to the knowledge of man. At times I would catch glimpses of something more, but it wasn't enough to make ground- breaking discoveries. I did the best I could with what I knew, and loved my patients to the depths of my soul. So many wonderful experiences occurred in which I will never forget- this was such a gift to learn and progress more.

Although I loved my work, with each child I bore, I experienced postpartum mood changes, still not as bad as the first. I had determined that taking medication was the best thing for me to do at that time, and frankly I didn't know anything else. I never looked outside of the sphere of Western Medicine. I loved being a mother, and I loved my children, and did my best to seek out positivity despite feeling down, depressed or dark. These postpartum mood episodes lasted between 6 months and a year. After my third child, things seemed to regulate again, but never back to where I felt that the switch was turned "off." I remember feeling distinctly like switches were turned on and off and I couldn't figure out what was causing the symptoms that were so troublesome. I never weaned off my medication from my last child. I felt dependent upon it to help me, in a way, and had a great deal of demands and stress in the various ways I was required to serve.

When my youngest baby was two, life was great. I had opened my own practice 5 years before that and it had launched me into an integrative mindset. I was willing to open my mind to new thoughts and ideas, and a lot of the integrative world resonated with me to be truth. The belief that plants and herbs God created were meant to help heal the body, and were designed by God for this purpose made a lot of sense. I started to incorporate natural remedies into my practice, while still administering prescriptions and providing treatment from a Western Medicine standpoint to those who desired it. I worked to develop intuition, knowing what would be beneficial for a patient, and what would not be helpful. I loved this period of growth and development, as it shifted me in a new direction and provided insight into the way God wants us to more fully heal.

In February of 2016, I was attending a medical conference when I started to experience strange symptoms. I began to have arthritis in my knees, trigger point pain up my neck, and headaches— all of which were atypical to me. I also had horrible insomnia and some anxiety again, and couldn't pinpoint what it was. Luckily at the conference during a luncheon, I sat next to a beloved colleague, who shared with me information about viruses and how they can cause a plethora of physical symptoms. While she did not know I was dealing with pain at the time, she was a heavenly messenger sent by God to deliver me with the truth of what was going on in my situation.

I immediately began to read Anthony William's first book about mystery chronic illness per her recommendation, and felt so much truth and light regarding this being a viral entity. Upon arriving home, I made appropriate shifts in my diet and started on supplements. I had never even taken vitamins before in my life! Immediately, I began to see improvement. I felt relieved that I caught this in time before it would become something greater. I also felt that my antidepressant would inhibit my ability to heal, and as I had experienced so much improvement — and now knowing the root cause of my mood changes were viral, I tapered off of it. It was an empowering feeling.

Life became a rollercoaster ride a few months into my journey. I had some good days, but more down days, and I began to experience deep depression. I started to have fibromyalgia and arthritis of my hands, knees and pain in my back. This was in the summer. After a few weeks, I prayed to the Lord to help me know what was needed for me to improve symptomatically. He indicated that I needed to give up grains in my diet. At this point I had already modified my diet significantly so this was another difficulty, but I obeyed. Within 10 days the arthritis and fibromyalgia were gone. I stayed on this course, continued with natural antiviral supplements, filled my diet with light through fruits and vegetables, and retained the optimism that I would heal.

Despite the difficulty of the way, I knew that my body could heal, as it was a gift from God and He had endowed me with power to overcome. Gradually, I started to improve. I went through moderate periods of anxiety and insomnia, but I persisted with the course. I didn't give up or look for other explanations behind my illness, and I remembered my witness that this was the path to follow. I chose not to look on the internet or entertain the ideologies of men. I knew I had received my answer, that this was viral, and I depended upon God to instruct me and guide me.

In December of 2016, I was feeling 85% better and very optimistic that I would be healed soon. I had stopped running in August of that year because I felt impressed by the Spirit that I needed to conserve energy and concentrate it on healing. This was hard, as I have been a runner the majority of my life (since the age of 12). Nevertheless, I was willing to give it up as the Lord directed me.

Despite my efforts, in January 2017, I started to get worse. More pains, but now they were burning and searing pains, sharp stabbing pains, boring pains and dull aches. I was not sleeping well at all, but I had learned to temper the anxiety about lack of sleep and would just lie patiently awake, thinking of positive things and images. I prayed for more faith in myself and more faith in God and in Christ, and more faith in my treatment plan. I clung to them, I yearned for them to be with me through this trial. There were points during this process that I cried out in frustration and heartache, but I never was angered toward God. I never gave up the hope that I could heal despite the extreme difficulty, pain, and exhaustion I was feeling. I never asked to be healed at this point either, as I did not feel prompted to. I knew there was a purpose to this trial, and I kept on.

In March, I became so weak, and had gone over a month with just a few hours of disrupted sleep per night. I ended up bedridden and unable to care for my children. I had to close the clinic down for a period. This was an extreme trial of faith, but I chose to trust in the Lord. I listened to uplifting talks, read scriptures and kept choral music flowing through my home. I would sit or lay in the sun for many hours a day. I felt drawn to the Sun, symbolic of the Savior and felt that He would help me heal.

I was blessed to meet with a wonderful practitioner, Muneeza Ahmed, who identified my condition as a shingles virus that was destroying my nervous system. I knew that I had a shingles virus, despite it never rashing and was taking supplements for it. I was told, however, that although I was on the appropriate supplementation, the dosage was not sufficient. I increased the amount, per her recommendations, and saw immediate relief- my sleep improved, as did my mood and energy. After four weeks, I was back at work and taking care of the demands of my family.

In July of 2017, I again had a dip, and continued to vacillate back and forth between feeling ok and feeling poorly. I still had not been able to run and it was discouraging. I started to experience gastrointestinal problems consistent with irritable bowel syndrome in February and although they had improved much, the symptoms still mildly persisted. I continued to have sharp stabbing pains that would come and go, as well as milder bouts of insomnia, but I persevered. I knew that my body could heal and I expressed faith in this daily, and conveyed it to my patients and their ability to heal as I served them. I found that during the days I worked to serve God's children who were sick, He would help me feel well. I was so grateful for that gift. Daily prayer and supplication helped me make it through this prolonged trial of faith.

Near the middle of August, the Spirit whispered to me, indicating that I had learned everything I needed to through this trial of faith, and that there was just one missing component. I was told that once I found this missing component, I would be healed and made whole. After a short period of time, I came to a profound realization. It was simple really, but I hadn't pondered it with the depth it required. I knew that my body could heal by God's power, but I had been depending on the supplements and the dietary changes so much that I was neglecting the power of the Spirit. In that moment, I knew that it would ultimately be God who would heal me.

I started to immerse myself in the scriptures. I had drastically cut out viewing media many months before and used that time, instead, to ponder and study, and do daily meditation. I would picture myself in the waters of Bethesda (John 5:5) and imagine them rising up over me, bathing me in light. I would imagine light coming down from heaven, coming through my head and down into my body, and I would send the light to areas of my pain and discomfort. I would lay on the grass and feel the energy of the earth and let it rise up and flow through me. Never before had I done meditation, but I was led by the Spirit with these images and what to do daily to receive more light into my soul.

I sat in the sun much and meditated about "the Son." I would picture myself as standing before God in perfection, full of light, and feeling His love for me. I recognized if I could see myself as He sees me, I would be made whole. I began to pray with more specificity-that I could have all barriers and blocks removed from my access to His power. This included preconceived notions, false beliefs/disbelief, or mistruths that I had been holding onto, as well as judgment of my fellow man. This shifting occurred quite readily as I allowed my spirit to be open to the Holy Ghost aligning me to God. I viewed myself as perfect in His eyes through Christ, and wanted to see that perfection in myself. I knew when that occurred I would be healed.

As the weeks progressed, I no longer felt as poorly. I even had a shingles outbreak on my hand, as a testament that faith in things which are unseen, but which are true— are still true. I started to have days where I felt completely normal, and I was learning how to alleviate my neuropathy and pain through the power of the Holy Spirit. I started to feel promptings that I no longer needed certain supplements. I continued to eat completely whole and natural foods to invigorate my mind and spirit. Shortly thereafter I was completely healed.

My healing came as a holy and sacred experience in the LDS temple. The Lord told me I was healed, completely whole and perfect before Him. It was because of my incredible faith in Him that this healing was able to occur. This miracle has felt like a dream to me, and I am certain it will take many years to process fully the significance of this great blessing. I am forever grateful for this trial of my health and faith, as it has brought so many significant and innumerable blessings to me even now.

God is omnipotent and wishes to give us *all* that He hath. But we are prevented from receiving these blessings when we believe that we are separated from Him or unworthy of His love, or that such blessings cannot be received in this life. We also limit ourselves when we believe that the power of God can only be accessed through others, or we are not allowed a portion of it to heal through the Holy Spirit. There is NO ceiling to gain access to His help as a child of God! He wants us to come to Him in a very real and distinct way, and He wants you to *know* and understand this.

Love is the highest power of healing. Without love of ourselves as God's creation, His love cannot illuminate us to the extent necessary to fully heal. This book is designed to help you feel His love, and open you up to more of His light so you can heal— and help others to come unto Him and be made whole as well.

CHAPTER 1

In the Beginning

"And the Gods formed man from the dust of the ground, and took his spirit (that is, the man's spirit) and put it into him; and breathed into his nostrils the breath of life, and man became a living soul."
Abraham 5:7

We each have been given the unique ability to experience our lives in the way God intended, that will create the most personal growth and spiritual stamina. This process is not always easy, but it is necessary for us to understand and learn lessons that can only be taught by the Spirit. It will be those experiences that allow us to return to our Heavenly home as a polished shaft, ready for further light and knowledge, and an increased capacity to learn.

In order to accomplish this grander goal, we needed to have a vessel that would allow us to feel things both physical and spiritual. It was a great undertaking, for our Heavenly Parents wanted to provide us with the best, most sacred and perfect vessel through which this could be done. It needed the ability to grow and develop in correlation with the phases of life and the passage of time. It had to age and decline so that our spirit would know when to leave it and return to our Heavenly Parents. It also had to be able to respond and adapt to environmental stressors and exposures. It needed the special ability to heal and recover from illness and trauma. Additionally, it needed to be connected to our spirit in such a way that every experience would be engraved in our sinews, to never be forgotten or discarded.

The pattern was set, and perfection was the purpose. Not a perfection that would be discovered in this life, but in the life hereafter, if we lived our temporal state in obedience to God's laws. Time and dedication spent on each vessel for each spirit was performed with the greatest love and consideration. Every detail was meticulously designed and formed, and we were involved in the process. We had chosen to come to earth, we had used our agency well, and this was the reward. Our bodies were created with love, and we loved them. We were grateful and excited to obtain them, and they were designed to love us back.

Our heart is the first organ that starts beating. This occurs at 6 weeks gestation, before our limbs are fully formed or even bones are calcified. It is the first place in which we can see life within the body. It is the centrality of our emotion. Our mind allows our bosom to burn when it is touched by the Spirit, our heart may skip a beat when we are nervous or excited, and we may feel a sinking heart when we are sad or betrayed. Our heart is vital to all other organ systems. Without it pumping 2,000 gallons of oxygenated blood daily, every cell in our body would perish.

The vascular system is the counterpart to the heart, and is in every way its own miracle. The soft, pliable walls of our arteries allow for expansion and recoil to accommodate the changing pressures with every heartbeat. The venous system allows residual nutrients to be recycled back to the heart for further distribution to the body, as well as to remove waste byproducts from the cells. This vascular system works in concert with the nervous system and responds to impulses from the brain when we are in danger or under stress. The objective is to provide our cells with essential oxygen and nutrients when it is needed most, and to prevent cell damage and death in times of crisis.

The brain is the manager of the body. It supports all other organs (like the heart and lungs) by its nerve pathways, which are connected to each of them. These organs transmit messages back to the brain along these pathways, telling the brain whether they are working optimally, or if they are diseased or dysfunctional.

There are parts of the brain that control breathing and digestion, as well as our heartbeat. This happens without our conscious control, and provides us with this essential service daily, so that it becomes an easy blessing to forget. This involuntary support system allows us to think and focus on other aspects of survival, and promotes our ability to develop in other ways.

Other areas of our brain were created to allow us to experience taste, touch, sight, sound, and smell. This enhances our mortal journey and exposes us to the entire array of senses to accompany our learning experience. Further still, the frontal cortex contains billions of nerve cells specifically designed to allow us independent thought, and the ability to have agency. We have delicately intertwined in our hippocampus the ability to retain memories, thus building knowledge from past experiences that promote our future path. To accommodate for the complex emotions we would need to feel and understand, multiple hormones called neurotransmitters were created, affecting our sleep and wake cycles, our mood and energy, and our cognition. These same neurotransmitters work in concert with the immune system to alert the body when infection or inflammation is present.

The immune system is the incredible guardian of our souls. It includes our spleen, lymph nodes, bone marrow, and thymus. It houses our white blood cells, which are made in the bone marrow and are our first line of protection when infection is present in the body. There are various types of white blood cells, which are specifically designed to mark new invaders, attack and destroy incoming threats, and remember previous infections. Additionally, there are white blood cells designated to clean up the postwar byproducts- whether it be dead viruses, bacteria, or toxins released. It is intimately linked to our neuroendocrine system (brain and hormone systems), with communication going back and forth between both areas constantly.

The endocrine system is our hormone-producing haven. It includes the master gland- the pituitary, which communicates from the brain to the ovaries/testes, thyroid, adrenal glands, and pancreas. These hormones regulate metabolism, energy production and expenditure, blood sugar regulation, menstrual cycles in women, fertility, fat storage and distribution. They help to decrease inflammation in the body produced by emotional stress, toxins, and infections. The adrenal glands in this system allow us to escape from danger, and produce adrenaline to prepare our body for "fight or flight."

The skeletal system provides structure and support to the muscles and ligaments, allowing us to move freely, with speed and agility when required. The ribs also protect our internal organs from trauma and insult. All bones start out as soft structures during fetal development, and become calcified when their internal formation is complete. They support a tremendous amount of pressure and the impact of walking, running, and virtually every activity throughout our lives.

Bones are flexible and more pliable in our younger years to allow for adequate growth and activity as children, but mature and harden with age. Within the bone marrow is the lifeblood. Billions of red blood cells are produced daily, to replace the billions that die off simultaneously. Iron is incorporated into hemoglobin to allow for oxygen transport throughout the entire body. White blood cells are produced in the marrow, to protect us from infection and inflammation. All this takes place quietly without our conscious awareness.

The respiratory system was designed to maximize surface area in order to obtain as much atmospheric oxygen as possible within one single breath. The windpipe, or trachea, divides into two branches that disperse the air into each lung. The airway further branches into smaller and smaller airways to allow the entire lung a chance for aeration and oxygen exchange. A mucosal barrier lines the entire airway, and it traps viruses, dust, pollen, mold and bacteria while allowing air to pass into the lungs.

The total surface area of the lungs is approximately the size of half a tennis court, and small, globe-like air sacs congregate at the end of the smallest branching airways. These alveoli are covered with capillaries, small blood vessels that diffuse oxygen into the blood and body. These delicate structures are what we depend upon, as well as the vascular system, to keep our cells alive.

The digestive system is formed from the same tissue that forms the brain in utero, and thus, often retains the name, "our second brain." It is the longest body system starting at the mouth, and continuing through the stomach, gallbladder, liver, intestines, and all the way down to the rectum. This complex system is designed to protect us from bacteria, mold or viruses found in the foods we ingest, while allowing absorption of the smallest micronutrients essential to our health and well being.

There are over 20 hormones produced in the digestive system designed to tell us when we are hungry or full. They also direct the breakdown and absorption of carbohydrates, fat, and protein, as well as vitamins and minerals. The bowel itself has more receptors for the neurotransmitter serotonin than the brain, and thus our gut can be associated with emotion as well. We may feel nervousness as "butterflies in our stomach," or nauseous when we are anxious or scared.

It is estimated that 60-70% of the immune system tissue is located around the digestive tract. The close relation and proximity is to optimize nutrient absorption and assimilation through the bowel. Housed within the bowel are over 100 trillion bacteria, which aide in digestion and assimilation of food. They also produce vitamin K and biotin, an important B vitamin for us to use. We could not survive without this good bacteria. They harvest the nutrients from our food and then pass it directly on to us.

These magnificent bodies were completed after a great deal of planning and preparation, and the final step was to produce a covering that would protect these incredible body systems. Protection was paramount, and God wanted it to also provide an external visage of beauty to match the beauty of our souls within. The skin is the largest organ of the entire body, weighing approximately 8-10 pounds on an adult, and is full of many miles of blood vessels. It allows us to maintain a very specific body temperature, prevents us from dehydration and infection, and initiates vitamin synthesis with the sunlight. It also permits us to feel the slightest touch of a fly, the coolness of falling snow, or the warmth of a fire. Additionally, it helps us to feel pain quickly and thus prevent further injury from external insults.

To support these divine structures, the world was created, a place whereon man could dwell and be proven herewith, to "do all things whatsoever the Lord their God shall command them." (Abr 3:25) The creative periods were formed and completed with the same divine dedication and purpose, based on what man would need to grow, develop and complete his sojourn on the earth. There was a division of light from darkness, night and day, to support man's need for rest and recovery, as well as work and productivity. A separation of the land from the many waters ensued, so that man could have a dry place to dwell and still obtain water to partake, to cleanse his body, and to cultivate the earth. There were seeds of all kinds placed in the soil, to grow fruits and flowers of all kinds, for the joy and use of man. There were placed beasts in the field, fowls of the air, and fishes of the sea in all their varieties to add beauty and diversity to the earth. All of this was completed through Jesus Christ.

"And it came to pass that the Lord spake unto Moses, saying: Behold, I reveal unto you concerning this heaven and this earth; write the words which I speak. I am the Beginning and the End, the Almighty God; by mine Only Begotten I created these things; yea, in the beginning I created the heaven, and the earth upon which thou standest." Moses 2:1

Thus flora and fauna were orchestrated for the use of man, and man was given dominion and stewardship over this vast and beautiful creation— with the inclusion of his *own* body. All things in and on the earth were created for the benefit of man in health and wellness, and for his succor and support in sickness. There was clean, fresh air for man to breathe, fresh fruits, vegetables and herbs to eat, and work for him to perform. The creation was complete, and now it was time for man to be introduced into the wondrous gift that was created specifically for him.

In the beginning, Adam and Eve were granted a special experience wherein they did not initially know good from evil, right from wrong, or joy from sorrow. They walked freely amidst perfection in the world, not knowing it existed; seeing, but not fully feeling, the love of God reflected in its blueprint. They did not know health from sickness, for there was no adversity yet to test or torment man. Nor did they know joy from sorrow, for they knew not how to procreate. Without physical increase, they could not have spiritual progression. These two wonderful beings were stuck in a perfect world without the ability to attain personal perfection.

After some time, the realization took hold, and Eve partook of the forbidden fruit. She did not do this with malicious intent, but out of selflessness to bring the rest of mankind to earth. I imagine Eve's decision was not done in haste, but with much deliberation. She knew that to partake of the fruit would bring life, but with it, opposition, pain, sickness and death. It would allow an adversarial force to tempt and try man in all his varieties, either to make them strong and resist, or to stumble and fall. Upon consumption of the fruit, her eyes were opened, and she had knowledge of the great plan of happiness.

"And Eve, his wife, heard all these things and was glad, saying: Were it not for our transgression we never should have had seed, and never should have known good and evil, and the joy of our redemption, and the eternal life which God giveth unto all the obedient."
Moses 5:11

She knew some of her posterity would fall prey to the evils of our day, and lay to waste their talents and spirituality. Yet, she realized that there was no other way for the great plan of God to occur, and within the struggle, could be found great joy and redemption. The partaking of the forbidden fruit occurs figuratively now, as each of us pass the veil and inhabit our physical bodies. That is where our personal mortality begins.

C HAPTER 2

The Ladder of Life

The beginning of Creation is spiritual matter. It is so fine it cannot be seen with the eye of man, but is the purest source of creation. It was present before the foundation of the world and we are all designed from it. Spiritual matter holds agency and can choose to form God asks of it. It chooses to obey His will because of the deep and abiding love it has for Him, and respects His immaculate consistency. This matter, once created spiritually, then obeys the laws and instructions in which it was set, and takes on physical form. It may stay fixed and firm to become a solid mass, or express fluidity to the likeness of water, or evaporate into the air around us. It obeys the laws of God and will remain predictable and true to its form, even when interacting with other elements. If it is combined with other matter to make something new- it will always remember and retain its identity.

The smallest unit of matter known to man is the atom. This is a representation of the universe in its vastness and glory, and is the pattern behind all the creations on earth. Each element and product is made up of atoms. Further still, the atoms can combine and coalesce to create molecules. Molecules then create other structures and cells. These molecules also form the ladder of life- the double helix, or DNA.

DNA was created spiritually prior to its physical incarnation and possesses a plethora of information unknown to man. The

9

length of the DNA is associated with the length of "life," or the information acquired by the individual. There is no "junk" DNA! Current research and science do not realize the wealth of spiritual information encoded in the double helix. Within the DNA are codes for spiritual gifts, talents and abilities, as well as life experiences and challenges that date back to the days of Adam. In this way, we are all connected to the beginning of the human family.

All the wonders of the earth were first created spiritually before physical representation took place. Plants, flowers, trees, shrubs, and all forms of animal life were also developed from spiritual DNA. It is their blueprint for learning and expression here on earth. The double helix also entails a representation of Heavenly Mother, Heavenly Father and Christ. One arm of the helix is Mother, the other is Father— and the central connecting "steps" of the helix is Christ, as He connects us together and provides the way back up to heaven. The amino acid bases from which the DNA is formed represent *us*, all the spirit children of Heavenly Father and Mother. We are all connected; we are all combined into one great whole this way. The bases for the DNA in its physicality were acquired from the dust of the earth, from which all things could spring forth.

As we are all part of the human family, we also acquire events and experiences that relate to the whole of human history. Covenants and contracts made with God by Abraham, Isaac and Jacob, are intertwined in the spiritual DNA of their offspring. God promised them each a land of inheritance, divine protection and eternal posterity as they kept His commandments.

Curses of Cain and the contracts he made with the adversary are also embedded in the spiritual DNA, as well as curses and evil contracts that other groups took upon themselves and their posterity. These produce animosity and opposition in our lives and among groups of people, and ultimately can prevent us from returning to our Heavenly Parents. The betrayal of Laban to Jacob, the barrenness of Sarai, the murders and fornications from biblical times, as well as their ripple effects, are all stored in the spiritual DNA and promote re-creation in our modern day.

Indeed, we see and feel the ripple effects of decisions made hundreds of years ago manifesting in society today, and these events are no different. We still have these spiritual and emotional wounds to deal with on a physical *and* spiritual level, and they are popping up more and more often in our daily lives. The frequency of such "gene expression" is increasing, to alert us of the necessity to *act*. We are here to change the expression of the spiritual DNA of humanity. It is upon each of us to silence and change the historical echoes that continue to create chaos in our world. We do this by utilizing the Atonement of Jesus Christ.

We are given spiritual and temporal traits that help us create our life. These allow us to grow, progress and learn as we experience the good and the bad, the joy and the sorrow, the light and the darkness, the pleasure and the pain. These traits are encoded and become part of the double helix as we come through the veil into mortality.

The blueprint of Godliness in its perfection does not include limitations of negativity, but we chose to incorporate them here in mortality so we could learn to overcome the natural man and turn to Christ. It was necessary for us to experience the vicissitudes of life that we could **know** the good from the evil. We could not *know—* fully understand and incorporate a concept— without it being woven into our sinews in a deep and abiding way. The double helix is the means by which this occurs. It is the path of the spirit into the body- the gateway is the mind.

Passage through the veil means forgetting our previous encounters to promote learning anew. Without the Spirit to lead the way, man would become lost and directionless. Therefore, in His mercy, God gave everyone the light of Christ. It is in the double helix, the representation of His life and love. This is a light that shines in the darkness, and cannot be uprooted from the body and spirit- for without it, they would cease to exist. It is the spark of divinity within us. The DNA is a testament of the love of Christ and our Heavenly Parents, and their hopes and dreams for us as their creations. Through it, we are intimately connected to the divine and all that is holy. We are children of a God! Because we have His light, we are given power to overcome ALL.

Inside the double helix are organized groups called "genes." Genes are smaller sequences of the DNA collectively programmed to produce the *code* for proteins, building blocks of life in the physical sense. In the spiritual sense, they are sequences of generations of time- lifetimes of knowledge and learning, compacted down into a smaller sum. In essence, it is like chapters to a book— one gene upon another, or one chapter upon another, culminating in the book of life. We are the book of life— it is the double helix.

"He that overcometh shall be clothed in white raiment, and
I will not blot out his name out of the book of life, but I will
confess his name before my Father and before his angels."
Revelation 3:5

If we can recognize the power of our thoughts, words and actions, as an actual representation IN the double helix, part of the book of life, we can proceed to make desired changes with the help of our Redeemer, Jesus Christ. In so doing, He will intercede for us, and our names will remain in the book of life as humble followers of our Lord and Master. Those who remain named in the book of life will not be cast aside, but welcomed into the presence of our Heavenly Father.

When information is acquired from a gene or "chapter," this is called transcription. Literally, the DNA "unzips" and a little copier molecule rides along one side of the DNA and obtains the genetic code for a particular protein. It carries this message outside of the nucleus into the outer part of the cell where it is then translated inside Ribosomes to become proteins, building blocks of life. Spiritually, the process of transcription is very similar. In order for the DNA to be copied, a promoter region- or the "start" section of the code, has to be activated. This promoter region represents faith.

Everything we do in this life is governed by faith, whether we know it or not. Breathing is an act of faith, because we trust there is oxygen in the atmosphere. Drinking water is an act of faith because we believe it will hydrate us and provide us with necessary minerals. We literally live by faith! The "copier" molecule is representative of our works. It is what transcribes or copies the "chapter" in our book of life, the double helix. When a gene or "chapter" is closed, it is due to a repressor situated on the gene that blocks the promoter region from starting to "write" or transcribe. A repressor can represent doubt or disbelief. When we do not believe something can occur, the gene or "chapter" of that particular experience will not be transcribed. We cannot access genes of our spiritual DNA when we express doubt.

When we view the spiritual DNA from this standpoint and the symbolism it entails, we further understand the phrase that "faith without works is dead." The message from spiritual DNA *cannot* be obtained without faith *and* works. Faith *is* work! Once the spiritual DNA has been encoded into messenger RNA, it is then taken outside of the cell nucleus to be translated. There, the messenger RNA is transferred over into proteins. These spiritual "proteins" are literally building blocks of our spirit- and the kingdom of God. We produce spiritual matter on a daily basis- whether for good *or* for evil. This is an incredible concept!

This process of spiritual transcription has deep symbolism. The messenger RNA represents messengers from God, delivering the "code" or true gospel of Christ to the human family. We are the human family. As we take the words of God into our lives, putting them into action, we produce fruit— Spiritual matter. These "fruits" or building blocks, in turn build the foundation of faith within us, heal the spiritual DNA of humanity, and help build the mansions in God's Kingdom.

"In my Father's house are many mansions: if it were not so,
I would have told you. I go to prepare a place for you.

*And if I go and prepare a place for you, I will come again, and
receive you unto myself; that where I am, there ye may be also."*
John 14:2-3

Our Savior Jesus Christ ascended to heaven after a dedicated
life of perfection so that we may know the path to follow and return
home. It is by following His word and His example that we are able
to transcribe our spiritual DNA via our faith and works, to translate
or "produce" building blocks of God's kingdom. Everything we think,
do, or say affects our progression.

All of the processes of life, survival and bodily functions, are
programmed into our DNA. It is the direction under which the
physical body takes form and function. It is pristine in its perfection,
but under worldly influences, physical strands can be broken or
damaged. Spiritual strands are never broken, but remain intact and in
place within the helix. Just as physical death or disease may temporally
separate us from loved ones, we are still connected spiritually.

The double helix thus also represents generational influences and
linkage. This is how belief systems and ideas can be passed down from
generations, including character traits, habits, etc. It is spiritually
done and set into the DNA. These belief systems can be good or bad,
and affect our view of the world around us, and our interactions with
others. We are required at times to be a "chain breaker" and heal the
ladder of life through spiritual rebirth and reformation. Seeing the
truth in all things and aligning to God's laws and **not** the ideas of man
are necessary for this alteration to take place.

When people break out of the poverty cycle or the cycle of
abuse— they are healing the double helix, turning it toward Christ
and making negative generational influences cease to express
themselves. Family history work thus takes on new meaning and can
help us to heal links in the chain (negative experiences or emotions)
that require freeing or liberation from captivity. In so doing, we help
the double helix to turn towards perfection in Christ. Our spirits do
this at the cellular level within the nucleus and directly in the DNA.

It is remarkable that such small and simple things can bring about such great changes in our physical state.

"Now ye may suppose that this is foolishness in me; but behold I say unto you, that by small and simple things are great things brought to pass; and small means in many instances doth confound the wise."
Alma 37:6

Thus, the small and simple changes we make everyday to turn toward Christ can alter our DNA expression in a big way. The more we incorporate love and light into our thoughts, feelings, and actions, the more light we will transcribe into our DNA. Our chapters will be full of hope, joy, faith, and love and we too, will be filled with these positive emotions.

Negative emotions and experiences can also be healed, and love can abound, when we work on the double helix through the power of the Holy Spirit. We have been given dominion over all things- and our own DNA is part of this! What a wonderful realization of this concept. As children of God, we are given guidance to find His truth and become changed through His Son, Jesus Christ. In His gospel are all the tools necessary to turn mediocre or flawed "chapters" of our DNA to perfection. Our lives can profoundly change when we are invested in this process to shift our DNA to light.

Prior to this mortal life, we helped create the components of our double helix. Through the thoughts, feelings, and actions we obtained prior to this existence, we created genes or "chapters" of our life, or sequences of time lived. These chapters then code for experiences, trials, challenges, gifts, and attributes, to be displayed in physical sense. We chose different things to learn and incorporate into our premortal life, and thus each individual's progression, talents, abilities and knowledge is different. We also each had the opportunity to learn the gospel of Jesus Christ, amongst other knowledge, prior to coming to earth. It was by our testimony of Him that we overcame the power of the adversary, who persuaded many to follow him instead.

Those who chose to follow Satan did not receive mortal probation- but are allowed to dissuade us from completing *our* mortal missions here on earth. We can choose to overcome his deception *again* in this physical state- by fortifying our testimony of Christ.

"And they overcame him by the blood of the lamb, and by the word of their testimony, and loved not their lives unto death."
Revelation 12:11

We each have similar genes coding for physical proteins and building blocks of life, but there are other genes that code for unique character traits and abilities. These are dependent upon what we learned and experienced prior to this life. Additionally, there are some genes that code for spiritual gifts. These may turn on and off dependent upon our need for those gifts during times of service or times of trial. However, we can also receive an endowment, or special spiritual gifts from above. These are bestowed based upon our faith and love of God, our service toward His children, and the promises we make to serve Him and remember Him.

Endowments are given via acquisition of that "chapter" or coding, and contain spiritual gifts and abilities supremely beyond the physical realm. As opposed to the genes of spiritual gifts, these are always available to open and be transcribed based on the person's faith, works, and worthiness. Temple attendance allows the "chapter" of this information to be transcribed again so the remembrance of these blessings and promises can occur.

Genes are opened (via acetylation or demethylation), similar to keys opening and closing doors. There are multiple keys to open even more facets within the gene sequence. We can obtain keys to operate and open certain genes or "chapters" based upon what we learn in this life, and the covenants we are willing to make and keep with God. Thus we may have the gene (the encoded information) without all the keys to completely unlock its full potential and use in our lives. There are main keys (like a house key) and smaller keys (like keys to the rooms inside it) that produce more information and knowledge from the "chapter".

The double helix resides within the cell, and is centrally located. On the exterior of the cell are spiritual receptors that look like trees, with branches on each receptor extending upward and outward. Each "tree" is a receptor of emotion and experience. For example, the receptors of love encompass different branches for the different emotions of love: love of God, love of man, love of self, love of earth. The more these receptors are signaled, the more the affinity for that particular emotion grows. The more the affinity grows the more that emotion is signaled.

Encoded experiences produced by our heart and mind are received and then taken inside the cell to the spiritual DNA. These "fruits," or our works, then pass through the nucleus (the veil) and present before the bar of God- our own DNA. In a way, this can represent the entire plan of happiness.

> *"Ye shall know them by their fruits. Do men gather grapes*
> *of thorns, or figs of thistles? Even so every good tree bringeth*
> *forth good fruit; but a corrupt tree bringeth forth evil fruit."*
> Matthew 7:16-17

It is important to note that initially you may not see the "fruits," or results of your labors to heal, or that of another. Change from darkness to light or from sickness to health, does not happen overnight. It occurs because of the choices we make everyday that propel us in one direction or the other. There are individuals who may have light in them, but are being persuaded to follow darkness. Deception is often a lot of truth mixed within a lie. Yet, ultimately, these fruits produced from deception will show forth externally. Like an addiction, one can proceed forth for a long time hiding their works, but the consequences of their choices will eventually show forth. Likewise, we can have health, but make poor dietary choices, and eventually experience illness as a result.

We can try all we want to hide negative fruits from others— but we can never hide them from God. Everyday we are transcribing and producing fruits from our thoughts that transmit into actions and are tied to feelings. We cannot run away from this concept. It is a truth. Those who are striving to produce good fruits and turn away from darkness will be immeasurably blessed.

On the other hand, those who willingly choose to diminish, belittle, or control another, are drinking damnation to their souls. Individuals who are spreading darkness and disease through their actions will have to stand before the bar of God. They may escape the physical plagues of our day, but they will not escape their judgment in the hereafter. Their soul will be in torment as they see the fruits of their labors placed before them.

Those who strive to transcribe fruits into light everyday will be added upon. More blessings and glory will be given, and they will receive the fullest measure of joy. If you feel like you have some negative "fruits" that need to be discarded, have no fear! The way is prepared, and we will discuss it in the following chapter.

Negative emotions can produce their own fruits— selfishness, judgment, dishonesty, betrayal, deception, and injury, and thus influence negativity in the world around them. We must have access to both ends of the emotional spectrum to fully learn. It is an incredibly important purpose for our learning in mortality. There must be opposition in all things.

"For it must needs be, that there is an opposition in all things. If not so... righteousness could not be brought to pass, neither wickedness, neither holiness nor misery, neither good nor bad. Wherefore, all things must needs be a compound in one; wherefore, if it should be one body it must needs remain as dead, having no life neither death, nor corruption nor incorruption, happiness nor misery, neither sense nor insensibility."
2 Nephi 2:11

The more we allow the positive emotions and experiences to flood the receptors, the more the receptors of negativity will diminish. They will wither and lose their potency. When the darkness is diminished from our bodies, we will experience symptomatic improvement with our illness or disease. As we continue on God's path to healing, incorporating more faith, hope, love and light, we *can* be made completely whole.

There are innumerable genes, or "chapters," as previously discussed. Some code for simple emotions, and others code for complex experiences. These are embedded in the DNA and they can be turned on or off, according to our thoughts, actions and beliefs. As the fruit of the experience presents before the DNA, it can incorporate the fruit and turn on gene expression. DNA has a natural affinity to shift to the positive, if we allow more light and love into our life. We have to do the work to turn on those spiritual genes and help them turn toward light (God) and shut off the darkness.

Like an electrical panel with breakers, the more breakers we turn on, the more light we can access in every room of our house. The more light we have on, the more darkness cannot remain. Casting out the darkness of fear, doubt and negativity, through Christ, is God's way to eliminate disease. God's will is that we BE perfect as He is— He wants to heal us and remove darkness of doubt from us by His power. This is done by Christ's sacrifice, which will be discussed in more detail in this book.

Indeed there will be times when we need to experience illness, and trials in order to grow and progress. We have to experience darkness in order to appreciate the light. But often, the gene or "chapter" encoding that experience is turned on for far too long, and we suffer needlessly. God wants His children to learn how to streamline the process of healing- spiritually, emotionally, and physically. He wants them to develop **real, true faith** in Him, to the extent they can heal completely! That is the purpose of this book.

God loves each of us, and He sees us as perfect *in* Him. This means we must work to be *like* Him. He wants this to occur, and intentionally turning the DNA expression towards His likeness expedites this process. The ability to turn on and off the DNA is granted to us through the power of Christ's Atonement, via the Holy Spirit.

How many times does scripture encourage us to turn unto Christ and cast away our weaknesses and errors? This becomes a very real process, which is done spiritually through the ladder of life. We need to turn on the genes of positivity and light, and silence or turn off the genes of negativity and darkness. Things we perceive as "hereditary conditions" do not need to be part of our life experience unless we choose it to be so. We can turn away from ancestral curses and contracts made with the adversary in the spiritual DNA and remove them, both personally and collectively, through the power of Jesus Christ.

You can ask God to help you shift the *altered exposition* coming from spiritual DNA that can contribute to the darkness of the soul and bring illness into the body. He may require work on your part, and direct you through specific actions through your faith. Following His guidance will silence the negative transcription from them.

We do not need to fear our future. This knowledge of epigenetics on a spiritual level is incredibly powerful and peace giving. It allows us to gain greater dominion over our very cells and the expression of our DNA. Ultimately, it allows us to access spiritual gifts, talents and abilities that can be granted to us in our time of illness to better manage through it.

The accession of these gifts is directly related to our faith in God and His power, and the use of the Holy Spirit to make the changes. It is actively seeking ways to promote these spiritual gifts in our external surroundings. If one wishes to develop the gift of charity, asking in faith to turn on those gene groups will be helpful. But one must also *act* on that desire to make the gene expression fully manifest itself. Faith is action— thus performing acts of service and striving to be kind and patient will help you develop the many gifts and facets of charity. You may also ask for the gifts or genes of kindness and patience to be activated to help you in your efforts.

It is like a small seed that is planted and nourished. The small seed of charity springs forth and grows into a tree which blossoms on the surface of the cell, with more receptors branching off for the expression of charity in innumerable ways. The genes within the DNA are then able to accept a variety of fruits, or encoded experiences of charity, from that receptor. It can then increase the reception of light into the DNA.

Conversely, negative emotions, such as fear, likewise can grow and form receptors on the cell surface, bringing fruits of darkness. It is important to note that fear, doubt, depression, hopelessness, confusion, and worry **are** of the adversary. He is very real, and is present on this earth with his minions. He will strive to discourage us from following truth, *every* step of the way. He will tell us that we are unworthy to save, that we aren't good enough, that we can't win, or would entice us to judge another. Often, the judgment we have of another is a demonstration of something within ourselves that needs work.

The adversary often will enshroud a cluster of truth within a small lie, making it seem right and good, but have a falsehood at its core. This confuses many on their path to find healing, who begin to vacillate among differing opinions and ideas. He wants us to remain sick! When we are ill with physical, spiritual, or emotional struggles, we are inhibited from looking outward to serve another, to better our communities, or to help our family. As illness and disease spread, our communities suffer because there is no one to stand up and serve. Families become divided and divorce ensues from financial distress, emotional burnout, and the disconnect that occurs with chronic illness. It is a cunning plan of the adversary, to deactivate our faith and trust in God through the spread of rampant illness.

Personal suffering is horrible, and collectively it is catastrophic. Yet we can overcome the wiles of the adversary by rising above the negativity with the help of Christ. We can work to control our thoughts and actions and strive to be loving, patient and peaceable. We can follow His example, ask for forgiveness from our errors, and be empowered to overcome from above. We can thus be protected from adversarial attacks! This will happen to the extent that we let God's complete truth into our lives.

"Thine hand shall be lifted up upon thy adversaries,
and all thine enemies shall be cut off." Micah 5:9

As we go about our day, we can choose how to manifest these emotions on the cell surface, and thereby influence the expression of our DNA. When there is more darkness, or negative emotions, in the body than there is light, we are prone to sickness or disease. We can find difficulty recovering from illness. As we add more light, or positive emotions, to our body, we can heal and overcome the physical trials of mortality.

You may wonder about the person who is always full of positivity and light- and still gets sick. At times we need humility, or to be grateful for our state of health. We are often given trials of health as an *invitation* to prove our dedication to God, to strengthen personal communication with Him, and adhere with *exact* obedience to *His* guidance in order to heal. There is more than one reason we experience illness in this life.

A virus, in spiritual terms, is a collection of beliefs or ideas adopted once in time by a group of people. These beliefs may be positive or negative, but both types of "viruses" serve a purpose. Negatively charged viruses bring the challenges of physical affliction or emotional turmoil. Some are designed to create chaos of the soul. Other viruses are positively charged, and help to fill us with hope, gratitude and love.

Both of these types of viruses can be created in real time based upon the beliefs of the people at present, or they can be historical viruses from previous chapters of life. Some of these viruses pass through generations. Some of them may never awaken to procreate and are silenced, while others can activate for a variety of reasons. Sometimes viruses will activate due to the individual's choosing- it was part of their desire in mortality to learn lessons through this specific process. Other times, these viruses can be activated by the energies around them, or further deceptions introduced into the body. They can sense negativity or lower energy and choose to activate as a result.

No one is ever going to escape catching a virus in their lifetime— it is part of the plan. Some viruses will be quick to clear based on the state of health of the individual (more light vs darkness, more positivity over negativity). This is why the connection between optimism and quicker recovery is scientifically noted. Other viruses may take root and slowly grow over time, imperceptibly causing mild symptoms until it suddenly severely attacks- creating a prolonged period of suffering and slower recovery. These are the darkest belief systems and ideas that are not easily uprooted (like secret combinations) and may take more pronounced measures to bring light back into the soul and drive the "virus" or belief system to dormant status. While the circumstance of chronic illness is difficult, it is a supreme opportunity to grow exponentially, unlike any other.

The current situation of our day is contributing to sickness of the body, mind, and spirit. We are enveloped in a world that is focused on frivolity, immediate gratification, and sensual desires. Almost everything is being taken from its purest form and watered down, or processed into something indistinguishable from its whole source. For example, processed foods contain little to no light, and have fractured spiritual attributes in them. Whole foods, particularly fresh fruits and vegetables, are loaded with light, and possess many more spiritual attributes such as gratitude, hope, and love. But whole foods are often not consumed readily, and even when consumed, it is not done with intention. This is a precious missed opportunity to add more light into our soul!

Gratefully, we *can* pray with intention. We can ask that the food we prepare bring us more love, light, hope, faith, or any attribute we are in need of. These will be absorbed from the food and latch onto cell receptors to flood the DNA with light. We can ask that any negative resonance be protected from our body and remain in the digestive tract to be excreted. Truly in whatever circumstance, if you do not have the means to eat as healthy as you'd like— praying with this intention is very powerful.

God knows when you are *truly* making the effort to heal, especially during those times when you do have access to healthy foods, and utilize them to your advantage. The process of healing is an *active* one and takes personal responsibility. We are ONE with God in this respect. We must do all we can to demonstrate our desire to be made whole on a physical, emotional and spiritual level. In order to receive *all* that God hath, including miracles of healing, we have to give *everything* we have— our might, mind, and strength— as we pursue the path to healing spiritually, emotionally, and physically.

"I, the Lord, am bound when ye do what I say, but when ye do not what I say, ye have no promise." D&C 82: 10

God is bound to bless us when we do what He says, and do *not* deviate from the true path to healing. But when we do not pursue this path to healing with diligence and drive, we cannot expect a miraculous recovery from chronic disease.

In addition to our thoughts, the programs that we watch on television really do matter, and actually affect our own programming! The beliefs, words, and actions viewed and heard on TV, the internet, Facebook, movies, or other forms of media, inform the mind and can create ideas, beliefs, and emotions. Dependent upon what we see or hear, we may create false beliefs that then make their way to the receptor of the cell and spread doubt into the double helix.

This is why praying for all the genes of discernment to be turned on and fully functioning is so essential. Many deceptions in the world about health, healing and well-being are preventing millions of people from accessing the true power to heal and overcome disease. In order to truly heal, you have to find the *truth* behind your illness in the physical, emotional or spiritual sense. Then you must incorporate the correct modalities God directs you to, so you can fully heal.

To heal takes *work*. I cannot underscore this enough. The personal responsibility to change your diet, incorporate exercise, or take certain supplementation is often essential to true healing. Unfortunately, our society has molded a medical system wherein most individuals desire a quick solution to their health problem, with very little accountability or responsibility. As such, modalities are incorporated which do not treat the underlying cause of the disease process, and merely manage symptoms. This does not bring true healing, and moreover, if the root cause is not addressed, darkness and disease will continue to spread in the body long term.

Thus one disease process can form another problem over time when not fixed. To incorporate a "quick fix," at times, is urgent and necessary. But we should always be aware that there is a greater underlying cause to address based on our symptoms, and we should not treat symptoms only. As we work towards this goal of healing from the root cause of illness, we will be greatly blessed.

Moreover, due to the divisive beliefs of the nation, we are inviting more negative viruses in, and more immune dysfunction is resulting. The general belief that we are safe, and do not need to prepare for war or disaster, deactivates the immune system. There are particular genes (warrior genes) that encode all the immune modulating agents— white blood cells, inflammatory cytokines, leukotrienes etc. If someone does not believe in fighting to protect their religion, rights and family, these warrior genes may be partially turned off. As we make the choice to turn these on by changing our present day belief system, we can help activate our immune system and bring it to full function. We may or may not be required to fight physically in this life against an adversary—but we all are in a battle of the spirit. Starting to win your own personal battle with the adversary, through Christ, is where the victory begins and healing comes.

The power of thought cannot be underscored enough. As a man

thinketh, so is he. The mind is where ideas form and coalesce to create a conceptual framework from which we compose our life's work— the chapters of our book. We envision from our mind, connected with the power of our hearts. If our heart's desire is the treasure and vain things of the world, our thoughts will feed into this. It is important that the mind and the heart are aligned to God. We cannot serve two masters, and it is imperative that we decisively make the split from the adversary now.

> *"As the plant springs from, and could not be without, the seed, so every act of a man springs from the hidden seeds of thought, and could not have appeared without them. This applies equally to those acts called 'spontaneous' and 'unpremeditated' as to those which are deliberately executed. ...*

> *"In the armoury of thought he forges the weapons by which he destroys himself; he also fashions the **tools** with which he builds for himself heavenly mansions of joy and strength and peace. ... Between these two extremes are all the grades of character, and man is their maker and master. ... Man is the master of thought, the molder of character, and the maker and shaper of condition, environment, and destiny"* (As a Man Thinketh [1983], 7–10).

> *"Let a man radically alter his thoughts, and he will be astonished at the rapid transformation it will effect in the material conditions of his life. Men imagine that thought can be kept secret, but it cannot; it rapidly crystallizes into habit, and habit solidifies into circumstance"* (As a Man Thinketh, 33–34).

How do we master the mind? By working everyday to change thought patterns. This cannot be done alone. We must do so by asking for help from above, and believe in God's power to help us. Notice how many times the adversary gives you negative thoughts in your mind. Recognize how dark and down it makes you feel.

How often do you think positive, optimistic thoughts? Notice how the positivity radiates happiness and joy from your soul. Learn to recognize the voice of the adversary and ignore it. The more you ignore it, the less present it will be in your life.

Personal meditations and pondering God's words bring more positivity into our mind, which then resonate with our hearts. We can change the thoughts of the mind and intentions of the heart more quickly by actively choosing to treasure up the true words of God through scripture than any other book. This takes our agency—our will. So often, we allow ourselves to be pulled down in thought, and we dwell there and allow more negativity to coalesce. However, we have the choice to rise above, even despite the difficulty. We are granted tools in this life to help us with this process, but ultimately it is *our* agency and our choice whether we will rise above or sink below the threshold of joy.

Remember the adversary is allowed to try us, to bring depression and doubt into the world. We can recognize his lies for what they are and cast them off! As a child of divinity, we possess the ultimate potential to overcome his lies and receive greater blessings for so doing. He cannot keep us down for long— we have the power within to break free of his influence through repentance and forgiveness.

It is important to note that there are pathogens and toxins in the physical sense that can create anxiety and depression of a clinical nature (William, 2015). These things spread darkness rapidly in the body and make it difficult to increase in light. Thus as we work to assist the body in removing the toxins and viral debris (both of which are resonances of darkness in a spiritual sense) and adding in more light through faith, hope and love, we can eradicate the darkness of depression in the body.

"Adam fell that men might be; and men are, that they might have joy."
2 Nephi 2:25

We are being pulled into a belief that joy is something to be sought outside of ourselves, that the world around us is the lens through which we will find it. This is a deception. Joy comes from within our souls as we connect to our Heavenly Father and recognize who we truly are, and the power we have to overcome with Christ. Joy will never be long term, constant, or purposeful if we are striving to find it outside of ourselves. This is a challenge we all face, to look upward to heaven for guidance and outward to serve, as we seek joy. Service brings joy. It helps us get out of toxic thoughts and plants seeds of kindness that bloom into treasured experiences. These memorable experiences can then carry us, and help us weather the dark storms when they arise.

It is also important to recognize that *your* belief is incredibly important, to increase personal light and obtain healing. If you don't believe that you can heal, or that a certain modality is going to help you, you will waste time and money and stay stuck in a mire of mud. Unbelief is actually a sin and will separate us from God. Thus, if you find you hold disbelief or unbelief in your heart, you will find it very difficult to heal. Start by asking forgiveness from your Heavenly Father so that communication between you both can open up. Recognize that He has placed many modalities and tools on this earth to help you heal— and a large portion of the efficacy of them will be your belief and trust that they will help as the spirit guides you to them.

There was a time in my life when I struggled with unbelief that anything could help me. It was a very hard struggle, and honestly, because of my unbelief, I did not see any relief with the medications I was taking. I had read about potential side effects online and was so afraid to take them. Therefore, I reacted negatively to them when I took them! As I had no other alternative at the time, I had to work to trust that they would work for me and help alleviate my symptoms. It was the only avenue known to me, but it was a great trial of my ability to trust— to let go and hand it over to God.

As I was able to trust that it would help me, and I worked through my fear, eventually the medication did prove to be helpful during that time. God allowed me respite, despite this not being the completion of my healing journey. Faith and trust in a modality are *essential*. Without faith and trust, you will find yourself at a standstill in your path to heal. Faith and trust in the *true* reasons behind your illness and the correct modalities to heal will bring you miracles!

Chapter 3

Acquisition

Like books in a library, the information recorded and stored in our DNA was obtained in a variety of ways. The majority of the chapters we obtained were based upon our experiences, and how we utilized our agency to learn and grow. God is merciful *and* just, and did not give us what we did not merit prior to this life. Some individuals were desirous to learn about music and art, others about science, still others became mathematicians. We each had chosen interests that drove the acquisition of our knowledge.

Imagine an endless library of information, wherein the truth of all understanding was contained. You enter the library and obtain all the books about a particular subject that you wish to study. This realm of study is far more creative than our current didactic learning on earth. Upon obtaining the information, it was literally encoded into your DNA— it became a chapter of your book! Additionally, you were able to experience the information visually, in a tactile format, and through emotional recognition. It became a part of you in a very real way, and following the acquisition, you "owned" the information.

This information, however, needed to be veiled, so we could create new experiences in the physical state. We seem to have no remembrance of these things, yet even now, we are drawn to certain topics of study, or naturally possess certain talents. This is because we've already learned these concepts in a spiritual sense, and are here to manifest growth physically.

Part of obtaining knowledge requires equal exchange. Just like an atom, one electron is shared with another, and then the other atom now searches out another electron. There is equal sharing between atoms, equal charges to balance the greater whole. We likewise shared information and knowledge with others pre-mortally. We had the opportunity to learn from teachers the mysteries of the universe, and were able to obtain as much knowledge and wisdom from these encounters as we desired.

Once we acquired this understanding, we were encouraged to teach it to others, thus providing equal exchange. As we each had the opportunity to teach and share our knowledge, the exchange of that knowledge could be solidified and improved upon in another way. As we shared information with individuals, we actually participated in creating and sharing chapters of our book of life. Essentially, a piece of our knowledge stayed with them, and their knowledge and experience was shared with us.

These experiences were also encoded in our DNA and it is why we often feel familiarity around certain individuals. There are times in our life here on earth when we will grow and learn something with specific individuals, and upon cessation of that experience, go our separate ways. A similar pattern emerged before this life, with interchange of information among individuals who shared a similar interest at one time. Some of our family members were individuals who had similar interests, or with whom we shared certain "chapters" in our life before mortality.

Before this life, there was an extremely long period of progression. We were encouraged to learn and develop talents, skills and abilities that would allow us to grow. There was always forward progression in the premortal world, but our desire and drive accelerated the pace. Additionally, there was information about God and Jesus Christ, and about others who would come to the earth to declare the words of God and encourage mankind to come to Him. All of this was available to us, and as we learned about many of these topics of study, we acquired knowledge. It became chapters in our book of life, coded in the way in which we experienced and perceived the information. Thus, even before we came, emotion and experience were part of our very being. Words began to form our ladder of life.

Another method of acquisition of our DNA library was based upon a "lease" of information, wherein we were allowed to "borrow" someone else's book or life experience. Literally, as spiritual beings, we could "read" the information of others, and experience what they had experienced exactly as they perceived it. Sometimes, we did this so we could understand another's viewpoint, or view the information in a different way so as to add to our own knowledge base. This was fundamental to our ability to understand our brothers and sisters, to develop empathy, and literally "walk where they have walked."

Those who had a keen interest in others prior to this life became empathic, and there are many who currently contrive this gift. Empaths are able to feel and understand another person's emotions even without the exchange of words. All of us, to some extent, are empaths. Dependent upon how we developed this gift, were the experiences we sought out before our sojourn in mortality.

The lease of information is how the Atonement of Jesus Christ was created. It literally was a DNA library of all of humanity, the imperfections and pain, sorrow, and suffering condensed into intense historical chapters that were transcribed in His very *cells* during His experience in Gethsemane and on Golgotha. This is truly how He was able to experience, feel, and understand everyone and their struggles perfectly, because the chapter of that individual was marked through *their* perceptions and understanding. He took on their emotions and experiences through their suffering and did not project His own experience into the Atonement. Thus He can understand each of us completely— He has read and understands everyone's book of life from their vantage point! How incredible is that? This is also how we are literally written on His very sinews, *never* to be forgotten. You are *never* forgotten. He knows your story, and it will always be remembered. It is also how He has obtained such *incredible* compassion and love for you.

"…Through the Holy Ghost the truth is woven into the very fiber and sinews of the body so that it cannot be forgotten" (Doctrines of Salvation, comp. Bruce R. McConkie, 3 vols. [1954–56], 1:47–48).

God has such love for His children that He often would bestow gifts from the library to each of us. This gifted information was granted unto us in love and delineated by what we already learned and experienced. We worked to develop these personal gifts, and they were granted to enhance our lives here on earth. They also gave us additional opportunities to evolve here as we proceeded to study and learn.

Thus, gifts of the Spirit are a form of acquisition from the divine library. Some of these gifts are the gift of faith, charity, hope, kindness, humility, service, patience, prayer and more. What spiritual gifts do you have? This is a fun exercise to ponder and write down any and all gifts that come to mind. You may be surprised with what comes up! Often these gifts may manifest themselves naturally. At other times, they need to be "unlocked" so we can access the information.

These gifts can be unlocked by pursuing experiences that would require their employment. For example, I truly feel that my health challenge was designed to help me unlock gifts of greater faith, patience, compassion, charity and service. I already had these gifts but they were underdeveloped until I was fully able to employ them due to my circumstance. I still believe there is more depth, even now to be developed through these attributes!

Many of these spiritual gifts can be applied to a large variety of situations. For example, one can develop patience with themselves, with God, with their children, with a neighbor, or with another family member. Thus the gift can be expressed in infinitely more ways than the initial designation may have been. We can grow the expression of the gift by working to obtain it in other areas of our lives.

We each had the opportunity to sit down with God prior to our mortality and go over our ladder of life up to that point. We counseled together to see what we had created and co-created, and what other things we wanted to experience in mortality. It was divinely orchestrated and we had the opportunity to discuss with our Father the additional things we wanted to incorporate. He, at times, would make suggestions, knowing our pattern and potential for growth here. We often would accept His suggestion about a chapter to be added— wherein, we could learn and transform into something new. Yet, all these experiences had been created spiritually by each of us before it would be manifested physically. These encoded experiences were stored in the spiritual DNA of humanity- our library of acquisition.

Similarly, when we read a chapter of a book, we may not recall word for word what the content was, but remember the underlying theme or emotion of that chapter. This concept also pertains to the chapters we live in mortality. They do not repeat over word for word, but there is an underlying theme or meaning to the experiences we receive. This is often why we keep having similar experiences over and over that relate to learning patience, or divine love— because it is the theme of a larger chapter.

Once we are able to learn the theme behind the chapter or experience, we are able to move on to the next chapter in the ladder of life and carry that knowledge with us. Truly, just as gene expression occurs on multiple levels and at the same time, we can be living experiences of a number of chapters at once. This is how we can build dimension upon a particular point of interest. For example, when an author starts out with one idea, it may be simple and direct. But then when the idea is applied to a variety of situations and circumstances, it blossoms into an infinite concept that can further develop and grow. Similarly, our lives allow us to draw upon a variety of chapters at once that then create a new and meaningful experience, all while tied to a foundational principle or theme.

In the beginning of our premortal life, we evolved mostly in love and joy. As time passed, however, and relationships evolved, individuals developed different ideas and opinions. At one point there was a war in heaven, which essentially was a battle among God's children. The topic of contention was acceptance and trust in God's plan for physical manifestation. This happened individually for each person, then collectively as one group, led by Lucifer, tried to dissuade the other group from trusting in Christ's ability to atone for us.

Many debated and encouraged their fellow brothers and sisters to consider the dichotomy of the two.

There came a division, and many rejected this plan of creation, agency and obtaining physical bodies. Lucifer wanted everyone to relinquish *personal* control of emotion and thought, and remove agency from the plan. Under his plan, everyone would be required to make the same choices and believe the same things; thus, all would return home unscathed. There would be no pain, hurt or heartache, as everyone would do exactly as they were instructed. His formulation of this earthly plan sounded enticing and logical, but it did not allow agency for free expression and thought, which would negate complete comprehension of our progress.

This process of debate did not happen overnight. It was a sequence of events the culminated in the final decision. It was during this period that many experienced sadness, sorrow, feeling abandonment, anger, frustration, and heartache. Many of those who rejected the plan were deeply loved by those who chose to come here and receive a body. This is often why fears of abandonment or codependency issues may arise in individuals even when they may not have experienced a temporal situation here that would trigger such behavior. They already experienced it once before, and are reliving the expression of that chapter.

Even today on this earth, we are reliving this battle as the adversary and his minions seek to destroy our freedom. Addictive substances, media, and products are created that promote psychological, emotional and physical dependence. They dampen our ability to break free of our own volition. We see it on an individual level, as well as collectively. It is a deception that creates control over others and

limits our understanding of the full purpose of life. We are meant to
act and not be acted upon. This is God's plan.

*"Wherefore the Lord God gave unto man that he should
act for himself. Wherefore, man could not act for himself,
save it be that he was enticed by the one or the other."*
2 Nephi 2:16

During my intense trial of health, as the sun would rise, there
were times I felt exhausted and disheveled. Many nights I didn't sleep
at all. Yet, the voice inside me said, "you choose— you choose." I could
choose to stay in bed and justify every reason for which I should not
get up and serve another, or choose to *act* and serve my family and
my other brothers and sisters, and ask for God's power to be with me.
Every time I made the choice to get up and do His will, I was blessed,
strengthened and given ability to make it through another day.

The more I sought to act in positive thought, action, and emotion,
the more I was able to overcome— one minute, one hour, and one day
at a time. There were times I was warned not to overextend myself—
and sometimes I didn't listen. That was when I became bedridden
for a month! Since that lesson, I have recognized His warning voice
when I am trying to take on more than I should. It is important we
find the balance in our lives so we can bless the lives of others, and
take care of ourselves as well.

To further understand the expression of words and emotions,
we must discuss spiritual energy. Energy is an unseen force to the
physical eye, but it is a foundation upon which all of creation stands.
There is a current of energy that runs through the human body,
giving it a life force and operating all functional structures. Without
this current of energy, we would cease to exist in this mortal sphere.
This spiritual energy of creation has varied frequencies and currents.
Emotions and words have energy frequencies attached to them, and
either can be positively or negatively charged.

When we are happy, joyful, and energetic, our energy frequency is elevated and the current of positive energy is flowing without inhibition through our soul. This brings in frequencies of light into the body. Light has energy to it, and there are vectors and wavelengths of it in varying degrees. The more light we incorporate— or the higher our energy frequency is maintained, the greater we will grow and enjoy emotional, spiritual, and physical wellness.

When we have gone through emotional upheaval, such as physical or emotional abuse, the negative emotions from that experience can literally create blocks of the energy current. The negative experience is transcribed into the DNA, and if we do not appropriately process the experience, we will continue to have that chapter open to us. It will continue to be read over and over, and more negative emotion will fill our soul. It will bring in more darkness, lower our energy frequency, and block the smooth current running through our body. This is how disease and illness can occur on an energetic and spiritual level.

Chapters of our books created by life experience, or drawn upon from the chapter of another (ancestral line), or emotions taken on by you from someone else in this life, literally can create physical manifestation of illness. When we are tired, depressed, and down— our energy frequency is low. The phrase, "bottom of the barrel" describes this perfectly. Our energy frequency can become so depleted through difficult experiences, or overextending ourselves that we feel we can't get any lower. We feel dark, down, and hopeless because the negative frequency is actually sucking out every positive expression from our life! Every emotion carries energy frequency with it, brings in light or darkness, and is the way emotion is expressed on a cellular, atomic level in the body.

Do you ever look at people who are always happy, and wonder how they stay so optimistic? Indeed, some of the most joyful and happy individuals I've met have not had an easy life. They are no different from the rest of us, but somehow they have learned how to let go of negative emotions and master the incorporation of positive experiences and perception. Faith is the foundation to this concept.

As we work to incorporate more positivity, we can create new experiences in joy and love, which then transcribe into the DNA. The more positive experiences we create, the more chapters for optimism we have to draw from in our personal library. And the more positive emotions we have being transcribed from the DNA, the easier it is to blot out the negative with the help of Christ.

Family history work can also allow you to identify individuals in your ancestral line whose chapter could be affecting *your* gene expression. A negative idea or belief adopted years ago may be perpetuating in your family line that is not healthy or helpful for anyone involved. Perhaps an ancestor committed errors that were grave in nature and their frustration, anger or sorrow is lingering within their chapter. Thus, learning of them and loving them completely can provide a witness to their challenges in mortality. When we feel a connection with our ancestors, it is because we acknowledge their chapters of life and what they went through. That can help them turn towards Christ to remove the negative transcription from their chapters. As this is done, we help fill our DNA with more light, and help our ancestors return to our Heavenly parents in righteousness.

"For the names of the righteous should be written in the book of life, and unto them will I grant an inheritance at my right hand. And now, my brethren, what have ye to say against this? I say unto you, if ye speak against this, it matters not, for the word of God must be fulfilled."
Alma 5:58

How amazing would it be if you found an ancestor who struggled, read their story, and validated the difficulty of their lives? Even more, how incredible would it be if you encouraged them to seek Christ on the other side of the veil, and you were privileged to meet them in eternal glory after this life, because they took your invitation? I promise there are many of our ancestors waiting for us to seek them out and witness their life! As we do so, we can repair the family ties in the chain that may have been severed in this physical plane. We can have the opportunity to live with them forever in the presence of our Heavenly Parents after this life. And in so doing, they can bless you with the power to heal! Indeed, many of our guardian angels are family members. They are empowered to help you heal if you do the same for them.

Chapter 4

Receptors and Reception

Our genes, or the chapters in our books of life, open and close, dependent upon the signals received by the cell. On the surface of the cell are millions of receptors, and many of them are unknown to science at this point in time. There are receptors for every single emotion we could ever possibly experience. These receptors have very high specificity— meaning they will only attach to the emotion and experience being produced at that very moment.

When we think of the emotion of love, the reception of love is far more specific! We can receive the love of a spouse in a certain way, or love of a family member as we talk over dinner. We can receive the love of a pet when we play catch with our dog or pat our kitten. All of these specific emotions of love have receptors encoded on the cell surface.

Similarly, we have receptors for negative emotions as well. There are receptors for anger of every manifestation, as well as greed, or envy or judgment of another. These receptors align along the cell in the opposite spectrum of the positive emotion. This again delineates the necessity of opposition in all things. It is as such so we may gain experience and use our agency wisely to choose well how we will react in every circumstance and situation.

It is natural to feel hurt or injured when someone does or says something negative to us. But we can heal from that experience by seeking out the light of Christ and having Him blot out the negative emotion from that experience. Doing so allows us to continue on the path of life in hope, faith, and love towards others. I recognize this is not an easy task, and it often takes time. But know that as you do your best to turn your chapters into light, you will be blessed and strengthened going forward. It will affect the future chapters you choose to create in your life! This is yet another reason why it is so important to work through emotional turmoil or pain as soon as you can. If it is not appropriately resolved in Christ, it will continue to follow you in everything you create.

Receptors on the cell surface are activated by the emotion and experience that is produced by the thoughts and intentions of our mind and heart. Through our agency, we control the thoughts of our mind, which feed into the emotions of our heart. The more we ponder upon the good things of this world, the more our hearts are filled with goodness, love, and hope.

The adversary will try to tempt us with negative thoughts about our self or others, but we have the power to choose if we will entertain those thoughts. The more we choose to think of positive and uplifting endeavors, the more positive things we will create in our lives. The more we allow negativity to enter our heart and mind, we create more of the same. The adversary will strive to keep you down and depressed, to encourage darkness and self-loathing.

Christ will illuminate your mind and heart with His light, help you recognize the divine potential you have, the child of God you are, and lift you up as *you* reach up to Him. The adversary will try to keep you inside yourself, forcing you to fight the battle of your mind on your own. He does not want you to look upward to God, or outward to help others, despite your difficulty. He wishes to keep you enclosed in a cage, feeling powerless to escape.

I testify to you that you can break free of the battle of the mind, of obsessive thoughts and depression. It takes work— a lot of faith, prayer, service, love, more service, and treasuring up the words of God so they can constantly flow through your mind. It starts with one minute at a time, then one hour at a time, then one day at a time. If you need medication temporarily to help, do not belittle yourself! But recognize the power within you to find the root cause to your symptoms and work on exercising the mind.

Little by little, encourage positive thought patterns to emerge, seek service in all things— opportunities to get out of your own head and help another. Pray for faith that you can overcome. Make this prayer a deep and abiding one, expressing the ultimate desires of your heart. The divine soul in you holds the desire to create in love, hope, faith and charity, and to propel your soul toward God. Your soul desires to transcribe positive emotions to *every* experience we encounter. The adversary knows this and will do everything in his power to bog you down and prevent you from experiencing joy.

As children of a God, our innate, truest desire is to encode the experiences of our life with *positive* emotions, even when the experience is difficult or challenging. We recognize that we are here to experience adversity, and that is what brings about a beautiful pattern of growth and development. When we can come to an awareness of this knowledge, and understand that our purpose here is to learn and grow, we can take on the challenges of life in a new way. We can see our illness as a stepping stone to develop more faith, determination, and spiritual strength, as opposed to a stumbling block which halts our progression. We can recognize that we are not left alone or comfortless, and that God's power is available to help us. We can recognize that the Holy Spirit can guide and direct us to heal from any and all difficulties through the Atonement of Christ.

> *"And I will pray the Father, and he shall give you*
> *another Comforter, that he may abide with you forever;*
> *Even the Spirit of* **truth***; whom the world cannot receive,*
> *because it seeth him not, neither knoweth him: but ye know*
> *him; for he dwelleth with you, and shall be in you.*
> *I will not leave you comfortless: I will come to you."*
> John 14: 16-18

How can we receive the Spirit of truth, the Comforter, without seeking *out* the truth of all things? If we are not ascribing to God's truth behind our illness, we cannot align to His paved path to a cure. We will be deceived and dissuaded by the beliefs of men. One degree off in our understanding of this concept can lead us down a prolonged path to healing. We can be carried so far away from the true source of information that when it is made known to us, we may feel unable to align to it. If we do not research all the modalities to heal from our illness, we will be unable to receive confirmation of which ones are right for us to follow. If we have tunnel vision of one modality, we could remain stuck for years until we recognize that we are not gaining any ground in our goals to heal.

We must seek out the truth, ask God to bring it to our awareness, and be open to receiving it, even if it isn't in the package we desired or hoped. It takes a willing heart and mind, and humility, to open up to God's truth. We will not be able to find **real** truth if we are stuck in a mire of half-truths or misleading information. If we truly desire with all our hearts to heal, and to seek the absolute truth behind our illness, it will be made manifest unto us through the Holy Spirit. We will gain greater faith, understanding, and power to overcome, because we will be aligned with God's truth.

Our cells have memory and will hold and store negative emotions when they are not appropriately addressed. This can create inner tumult and upheaval. Blocks can be created to protect our heart when it has been injured or forgotten, making it difficult to access emotions of positivity. Yet we can work through these obstacles by spiritual epigenetics. Striving to turn on every gene of faith in God and ourselves we can muster, then working to open up hope and love through service, and casting out the adversary in all His deceptions, will alter the spiritual DNA.

The brain, as the manager, is imperative. It records all the experiences we have ever had with emotions affixed, and sends the messages to the cells for DNA transcription. It has the choice to shift the emotion to light before transcription is complete, however. We have the agency to choose how we respond or react in any situation. The belief that, "we are just who we are" and cannot change, is a fallacy and does not promote personal growth and development. Emotion and experience are intertwined together, like two sinews bound. Thus experiences are triggers to emotions.

This is why, upon recalling a pleasant memory, the same emotions from that experience arise as you recall the experience itself— the setting, the time of day, the weather, who you were with, etc. This can also be a reason behind post-traumatic stress disorders and anxiety disorders.

When a very negative experience occurs in our lives and creates an incredible amount of anxiety, the brain records that experience and the emotion of anxiety tied to it. It travels to the cell receptors of EVERY cell in your body, and is transcribed by the DNA and encoded in the soul. If the experience happens again, it will also be recorded in the cell via transcription and translation. The cell retains the memory of the experience and the emotion that was tied to it, so it labels the experience again with "anxiety." Thus, it will open up the gene of that experience and emotion once more, and transcribe it all over again.

This is why flashbacks occur— because literally the spiritual DNA is opening up the gene or "chapter" from the previous experience at the same time as the similar experience is going on. Often, this is why the emotion for the subsequent encounter is stronger and more uncomfortable. This can also provide an explanation for why anti-anxiety medications and anti-depressant medications do not often provide long term relief. The experience and emotion recorded is in EVERY cell of the body, so when the experience arises again, it will be processed in a similar fashion in the cell memory.

Medications will affect the processing center— the brain— and they can dampen its ability to send the subsequent messages so that it isn't recorded with the same intensity. But the cells are smart, and they begin to recognize the similar experiences and thus attach them to the emotions for which they have historically been encoded— anxiety, depression, anger, frustration. The emotions will therefore begin rising to the surface again— a sign that something needs to be addressed. Often, all that is recommended is a different medication.

Counseling can be beneficial because this helps change cell memory and alter the thought patterns that were recording the negative emotions with the experiences. If psychologists and mental health professionals take it one step further, and see the benefit of healing via spiritual epigenetics, they will see remarkable progress. By developing faith and incorporating positive experiences, we can silence that chapter or experience. Even more so, we can incorporate Christ as our coauthor to help us rewrite the chapter, eliminating all the bad, negative and hurtful emotions from it. This is how the power of the Atonement works. It takes work on our end to change our thought patterns and behaviors, but as we show our desire to do so, we are blessed and He becomes the coauthor to our book of life.

If you deal with PTSD or anxiety, you are invited to try this exercise. The more faith in God and yourself you have, the more powerful it will be. Even so, continuing to ask in faith will always be helpful. First, ask if it is possible for you to be done with the trial of PTSD about (blank). If He says yes, then ask for genes of remembrance of that initial experience that caused the negative emotion to be silenced, and the triggers removed. You will receive affirmation that this will be so and you will start to see how the reprogramming is helping. You still must work to incorporate more positive experiences into the DNA, but it will become easier.

Every time you feel triggered by something, go back to the initial experience where it is coming from and ask Heavenly Father if you can silence that "gene" or experience, and remove the trigger. If you don't even know why you are triggered, you may ask God to help you identify it, or ask if you can merely silence the historical experience and remove the trigger to it. Often He will want you to identify what the issue is so you can learn from it and truly heal from it— have it blotted out of your book altogether. If you can't identify it immediately, however, asking in a more vague form may still be helpful.

As always, work to fill your life with new experiences and positive emotions. Interacting with nature and animals, or serving others, are powerful ways to add in positive experiences. God may temporarily silence the painful chapter for your benefit, or want you to address it directly by rewriting it with Christ to blot out the negativity. See what answers come to you.

Receptors can grow in affinity towards light or darkness—positivity or negativity. The more we flood our body with negative emotions, the more receptors are created to accept them. The same is true for positive emotions. The goal is to continue transcribing experiences in positivity so as to overcome any and all negative emotion through Christ. As we do this, the receptors on the cell surface for negativity are diminished by attenuance. When more positive transcription is taking place, the negative receptors decline in number. The adversary will *not* want you to succeed with this, so if you feel like negative emotions are heightened, keep pressing forward! With time and persistence, you will come off conqueror. We can overcome *all* things through our faith in Christ.

*Nay, in all these things we are more than conquerors through **him that loved us**. For I am persuaded, that neither death, nor life, nor angels, nor principalities, nor powers, nor things present, nor things to come, nor height, nor depth, nor any other creature, shall be able to separate us from the love of God, which is in Christ Jesus our Lord.*
Romans 8:37-39

At times, you may feel hostility towards your progression from an unseen source, and this could be from a member of your ancestral line who does not want their chapter turned or altered. They feel as if it will be an identity crisis of sorts. Indeed, as you change and adapt and improve, it affects the expression of their spiritual DNA as well. If you receive this impression, it is helpful to speak with them and let them know they are not going to be forgotten, and help them understand this process of turning toward more light. Let them know they are loved and this change will affect them and generations to come for the better. Often by doing this, you will feel peace as they recognize this truth and go on their way. This emotion/experience transcription cannot yet be seen with our current medical advances. It is a process done entirely by the spirit, but it will affect the physical expression of the DNA, which is under study today.

What does it mean to receive? A modern day definition is generally— to be given something. However, I desire to take this a step further. To receive requires personal *action*. To really and truly receive something, we must accept it with our heart and soul. Receiving instruction from God will not come if we are not willing to do something with it. If we receive a gift from someone and we never open it— then what is the point of the gift? If we never use the sweater, or the juicer, or whatever the gift may be, then why even accept it?

There are many different ways in which people receive things today. How do you receive constructive criticism for example? When faced with a challenge that magnifies your weakness, do you kick back in anger and frustration, or do you receive the challenge as an opportunity to grow and make the weakness your strength? How do you receive the inspired insight and intuition of others on your behalf? Do you immediately close down and trust in your own knowing, or are you willing to step outside of yourself and consider things anew? What do you do with new information you receive? Do you put it on a shelf for another day, or do you ponder its meaning and ask God if it is correct? If He tells you it is right, will you be willing to implement it into your life, even if it is a dramatic alteration in your previous ideology?

To *receive* is to be true and faithful in all things. It means a willingness to act and utilize what you are given. There are many, many gifts that God wishes to bestow on His children— but all too often, they are too busy to receive them. Or, they are numbed by worldly influences and opposition, and not even turned toward Him to ask what is waiting for them. For your cell receptors to be sensitive and ready to accept new information— you, likewise, need to be in this pattern of thought to receive. By doing this, you will reap the benefit of having a predisposition of more positive receptors on the cell surface.

On a spiritual level, we need to be able to understand messages we receive from God through the Holy Spirit. There are varied messages and promptings in the world today, but there are three sources from which we receive information (Pontius, 2014). The first source is the one we should all strive to follow— this is the voice of the Holy Spirit. The Holy Spirit is also known as our conscience— it lets us know between what is right and wrong. It helps to direct our choices in righteous ways and warns us of impending danger. The Holy Ghost also provides comfort to us when we are full of sorrow. It can purify us, cleanse us, and *heal* us through its light. The Holy Spirit's influence can empower every one of us to make the right choice and stick with it.

When we act on one prompting of the Holy Spirit, we will be given another. The more we follow these promptings, the more we will be led to God's truth in all things. We will have events occur in our lives that will testify of God's awareness of us, and His desire to lead us to more light and truth. He will meet us where we are at. He will give us the knowledge we are ready to receive and build upon. The Holy Spirit enlightens our minds, and quickens our understanding so we can move from one precept to the next, seamlessly building our knowledge with wisdom and poise. Usually, this voice comes to us in the form of our *own* voice, but sometimes it may be the voice of a man.

Sometimes, we may ask to receive an answer and it doesn't come immediately. It may take days, weeks or months to receive the answer— but it often will come with time and diligence. Often a word may enter your mind, and you may be encouraged to study that word, which unfolds more information and knowledge to you, and eventually leads you to your answer. Sometimes, your answer will come through another person. Sometimes, you may act on a prompting, and in the middle of it, feel like everything is a mess! That doesn't mean the initial impression was wrong. Stick with it and continue on your chosen path and you will see the fruits of your labors.

The Holy Spirit will tell you *one* thing to act on at time, from which comes another prompting or insight. It is *always* positive and good, and will bring good to yourself and others. It will make you feel joy, hopeful, and full of light. Be aware that the Holy Spirit will tell you in your mind *and* in your heart. Both are essential and cannot be discounted. The adversary can try and mimic impressions of the Spirit by sending impressions in your heart. You can identify this disconnect, however, as the mind will not coincide with the heart in this instance.

When *both* the heart and mind are aligned, and clarity comes to you, this is the Holy Spirit. There were times when I was told *not* to exercise, or do something that I desired. This was the wisdom of the Holy Spirit, knowing my physical condition and what I needed to do to heal. Be open to these impressions, even if they seem counterintuitive. If they come from the Spirit, you will be blessed to obey.

The next source of information is our own mind and thought. This part of communication is where we plan dinner, or the next grocery trip, or figure out a family vacation. It is typically filled with the daily tasks that occupy our time, and produce little change in the long-term outcome of our life. The differentiation can be felt between the self voice versus the Holy Spirit. The Holy Spirit will always inspire you and guide you to make changes— and give you challenges— to find, or stay, on the path that will accelerate your progression to God.

The voice of the mind will not give you truths of eternal consequence, but is meant to help you manage the daily tasks of your life. If you pray about work or where to live, and receive no answer, it is probably because neither will be of consequence to your eternal outcome. At times, you may feel impressed to change jobs or housing locations, and if you receive confirmation from the Holy Spirit, then go with it! At other times if you do not…it doesn't mean that you shouldn't make the change, merely that it is not of eternal import and either choice is fine.

The last source of information is a voice we should strive to avoid. This is the voice of the adversary— or dissonance. Often this voice will come *following* a prompting to do something good, and will try to dissuade you from acting. It clashes with the good intimations you receive. The expressions of "you're too tired," or "you don't have time," or "they don't need it," will deter you from acting on the initial impression. Your mind will be filled with all the negative, yet valid reasons why it isn't a good idea to exercise, or to go serve someone else, or to change your diet. *Especially* with your health!

You may feel inspired to go an entirely different way in treating your health condition, but then all these negative voices come in and make you feel heavy, weighed down and confused. Confusion is *never* from the Spirit. The Holy Spirit brings clarity. If you feel heavy, confused, or weighed down— you have an adversarial force at play. When this occurs, pray for more clarity, and work to listen to your heart and mind. Do not feel you have to act immediately, but let things percolate before you proceed. The Holy Spirit's voice falls readily upon those with patient ears.

The more you recognize and act on the promptings of the Holy Spirit, the more you will receive in understanding. It is essential to take this challenge—act on every prompting of the Spirit— to gain more light and knowledge, to understand the truth of all things, and to come at an accelerated pace to God and healing miracles. Obtaining the *gift* of the Holy Ghost through proper authority augments this progression and allows greater light to flow through you and into your life. Through this gift, we are no longer partakers of His mere influence, but *receive* the Holy Ghost as a constant companion through our worthiness. More purification and healing occur when we follow Spiritual promptings and make promises to follow the path to God. This is the ultimate reception, and a constant blessing in our lives.

Spiritual Epigenetics

Within the genome, there are a host of multiple functions at varying degrees and levels. Each one is specific to cell functions and needs, and is individually appointed. These genes can be turned on or off like light switches, according to the electrical activity of the cell— or the cell signals that arise from emotions and environmental influences. This differs from physical epigenetics, as the focus is often on just external influences, such as exposure to toxins and chemicals, dietary intake, and medications.

Spiritual epigenetics is the direct way in which the spiritual DNA is expressed through internal influences and behaviors, which are chosen by the individual to bring a thought to action— to fruition. When these genes are displayed in their ordinary form, they look inactive to the human eye. But they are transcribing millions of times a second, and are in complete harmony with the individual's frame of mind and heart at the time of transcription. Double stranded DNA allows for a variety of gene expression, as more sequences are incorporated into the genome of the individual. DNA strands represent the book of life— eternal experience, and a record of what has been learned and understood prior to this life.

It includes all the codes necessary to develop spiritually and overcome the natural man (physical body) through faith in God. DNA is not hemispheric and is a continuum of one great whole, one eternal round. It can change expression, dependent upon how our spirit interacts with our body. The more the natural man is suppressed, the more our spirit can grow to fruition and turn on more of the positive spiritual DNA. The more the natural man is accustomed to overcoming our spirit, the more these genes are diminished in their power and capability, and the more the physical DNA can take precedence in function and form.

Thus, it is imperative that the individual learn how to overcome the tendencies of the natural man— the greed, envy, hate, judgment, pessimism, and hopelessness. These are all adversarial measures used to negate the power of the Spirit over the natural man. We *can* overcome these tendencies— it is completely possible through our Savior.

> *"For the natural man is an enemy to God, and has been from the fall of Adam, and will be forever and ever, unless he yield to the enticings of the Holy Spirit, and putteth off the natural man and becometh a saint through the Atonement of Christ the Lord, and becometh as a child, submissive, meek, humble, patient, full of love, willing to submit to all things which the Lord seeth fit to inflict upon him, even as a child doth submit to his father."*
> Mosiah 3:19

Cultivating love for God, self and our fellow man allows the switches of spiritual DNA to be primed for access. These are primed via keys, keys of power from above by which the genes can be accessed for transcription. These keys are bestowed upon those who demonstrate their faith in God and have worked to gain knowledge and understanding of the virtues— love, hope, faith, charity, kindness, patience, long-suffering. When we are willing to give up the natural man, we do so with intention. We ask God to change us from a fallen state in a specific area— greed or egoism for example, and we work to change those tendencies in their manifestation, making our weaknesses our strengths.

When we are fully penitent and desire to continue implementing positive changes, the negative exposition may be silenced, and more genes of charity and selflessness are turned on. Thus we obtain more power, and grow the opposite emotion to overcome the negative ones in question. This is how spiritual epigenetics work. One cannot merely ask for a switch to be flipped— it is done by personal dedication to God's laws, and a sincere desire to be changed and turned in the right direction. As we pursue the work placed before us with a pure heart and real intent, we become a polished shaft of light. Literally, the DNA is changed and altered from its fallen form into perfection through Christ, to become those genes of deity.

Additional genes, or chapters of deity, can be spliced into the DNA as a new gift or endowment occurs. These are direct gifts of genes of the divine, and are usually given in response to great obedience and faith in God. Such genes will always be turned on thereafter and available for transcription, as long as the individual is striving to follow God's laws.

Additionally, there are spiritual gifts that can be temporarily bestowed in response to a need. When one is going through an intense trial of health, for example, one can specifically ask for genes of hope, faith to be healed, faith to heal, more faith in oneself, wholeness and oneness, and faith in God. These can remain on during the trial to help us heal.

It is important to understand— faith in God and in oneself is *always* essential for healing. These genes need to be accessed and transcribed first, before any other reaction can occur. Also, when a child is adopted into a family, spiritual genes are spliced in the individual wherein all the historical promises and blessings given to the family lineage will be now inherited from the parents into the adopted child. Literally adoption can create new gene splicing on a spiritual level, and affect physical manifestation of the DNA.

When we are infested with genes of negativity, the whole chain of DNA is affected adversely. These genes allow the dark emotions to spread along the DNA chain and contaminate its potential for purity. Negativity is disease promoting, and encourages the progression of illness. Fear is the inducer to negative genes, and the works created in fear transcribe codes for hate, anger, frustration, selfishness, judgement, self-loathing, and domination of another. All of this transcription goes out of the nuclear envelope into the Terasomes (spiritual equivalent of ribosomes). They translate the genetic code emitted from the gene and it produces building blocks— spiritual protein. These spiritual proteins literally build God's kingdom in heaven, and are based upon our works of faith. Works in fear will negate the works of faith and reduce their power to heal us and build us up spiritually.

> *"You can't, you don't, build out of pessimism or cynicism. You look with optimism, work with faith, and things happen."*
> Gordon B Hinckley (from *Ensign*, June 1995, 4).

Thus it is important to strive for optimism in all things, despite the difficulty of the way. One can specifically ask for genes of optimism and hope to be turned on, and can even specify it to be hope in oneself, or in God etc. The more we work for these positive emotions to become a natural part of our expression, the more they will remain on, transcribing words of light and love into our soul.

There are other factors that can affect spiritual gene expression. Experiences of abuse, neglect, being bullied, being an outcast, or feeling isolated will all impact the spiritual DNA in a very big way. This is not the individual's fault, but we can ask that Christ be our coauthor to eliminate all the negativity contained from these experiences. We have to be ready and willing to let go of anger, frustration and fear towards those who were involved in order for His healing to happen. Often due to the negative experiences, genes of mistrust, disbelief, and anger towards God are turned on. We can literally ask for genes of remembrance of the negative experiences of our life to be silenced, and the trigger removed.

We can also ask that genes of remembrance of positive experiences be turned on, that we may more easily fill our soul with positivity and light. As you do this in faith— and continue to show your works by serving others, you will feel a shift within you. A new brightness of hope and restoration of goodwill will flow into you, and you will be able to progress towards more faith and hope and love. It is remarkable to behold. Cells will retain memory even after the change, so if you still run into a couple hiccups along the way, do not be alarmed. Hold fast in faith and know that these changes are taking place, and will remain permanent, according to your diligence.

There are other genes that can pull us down in our frequency. Genes or "chapters" of despair, doubt, dismay, disillusionment, depression, confusion, or divergence can also be turned on by our thoughts and actions, and thus create negativity or darkness in the body. Some of these genes are not even from our own doing in this life, but are from historical beliefs and experiences! Thus it is wise to recognize that familial lines may carry "chapter baggage" that needs repair in the ladder of life.

Cancer is caused by inappropriate cell division in which the DNA sequence has been improperly copied and divided within the cell. Therefore, the code becomes jumbled, and confusion and chaos ensue. The cells begin to multiply rapidly because the negative transcription phase has no holding pattern— it is no longer functioning under the divine law of "filling the measure of its creation." It thus encroaches upon other organs and tissues that are not receptive to the new cells. Some of these cells will be infected with the "false message" and begin production of more of the same.

Cancer begins, in a spiritual sense, when a viral body (negative belief system once adopted by a group of people, like a secret society) feeds upon toxins that emit greed, envy, or lust. These emotions (or toxins in the physical sense) fuel the negative belief system to then grow and multiply to the extent that there are not enough regulatory genes to prevent overexpansion. The negative beliefs, essentially, overtake the good spiritual genes, silencing them, or taking them hostage, to carry out their pursuits.

Everyday, each of us has some form of cancer cells. It is imperative to include light through our dietary choices and attitudes, and reduce environmental exposures to toxins. But we can also encourage these aberrant cells to be squelched by turning on the warrior genes of light (our immune system), and have them specifically trained to the virus causing the negative transcription. We can ask that all cellular "hostages" be released, and the debris of battle contained and exhumed. Thus in a spiritual sense, the cancer cannot fester and grow. We can also ask that the genes of resolution and repair be turned on to help remove the dead debris and toxins that will produce more of the same if they remain in the body.

I realize that these are all new concepts. But, remember, we are literally spiritual beings first, in a mortal sphere. It is time we start recognizing this, and treat disease and illness from a spiritual perspective, according to God's will— that we learn The Healer's Art. He has *all* power to remove and rebuke any illness or disease, if we have enough faith and trust in Him. His power can overcome any illness, disease, or plague set upon us, despite the beliefs of men. Obedience to His will brings blessings, but *exact* obedience will bring miracles of healing.

> *"Yea and they did obey and observe to perform every*
> *word of command with **exactness**, yea and even*
> *according to their faith it was done unto them..."*
> Alma 57:21

This scripture referenced above is in regards to an army of two thousand inexperienced adolescents who went up against a huge army of well trained and war weathered men. They did not fear death, and they knew God would protect them in battle. The miracle was that because of their *exact* obedience, not one of them died, and they won victory over their foes! So it can be with us— we can be victor over our health challenges as we make all the necessary changes, and consistently stick with the plan we are inspired to follow, taking it one day at a time.

Another extremely important factor is how we care for our bodies on a spiritual and physical level. When we exercise for example, we are not only boosting our cardiovascular health, but we are activating warrior genes. They are exercising along with us, if you will, producing natural killer cells, lymphocytes, and other white blood cells, to patrol and cleanse the body. We, additionally, are perfusing the tissues and cells with oxygen— a principle fuel of life. This oxygen has not only a physical benefit, but many, many spiritual benefits with it. Essentially, it gives us more faith and endurance to overcome and withstand any spiritual and physical difficulties that beset us.

Isn't it interesting that we cannot see oxygen, and yet depend upon it for our existence? God is like oxygen— for without Him, we would all perish. This is also why deep breathing is so beneficial. You deeply oxygenate the tissues and perfuse them with more light as you deep breath. It is even MORE beneficial to meditate while doing this exercise, imagining the expelling of all the negative emotions, frustration, or stress. Similarly, you can just imagine expelling darkness— and breathing in light, love, hope, and charity. Literally, when we do this, those very negative emotions will be exhaled out of our body and allow light into our frame. Whenever we want to incorporate positive emotions, we need to make room for them! Thus looking for ways to move out the negative experiences and emotions are essential, and deep breathing is one of many ways to do this.

Food is essential to life, and all food has spiritual power within it. When food is in its natural and whole state— it's perfected form as God designed it— it has many more abilities to lift us and fill us with light. Unaltered fruits and vegetables are infused with happiness, joy, faith, hope, love, and light. They grow in gratitude in their surroundings, and when we grow it ourselves, the nutritional content is specifically designed for us and our needs. Literally, the spirit of the plant interacts with our own, and can calculate what our nutritional needs are!

It is amazing how much love and gratitude can be felt from whole foods. We will always receive some of these spiritual blessings when we ingest whole foods, but we can capitalize on their consumption when we pray and ask specifically to absorb more love, hope, faith, gratitude, or whatever we need, from the food and give thanks for it.

We will then have receptors for those qualities and characteristics line our digestive tract and pick up on all that is positive.

Processed and genetically modified food is not what God intended us to eat, and is a diversion of man's creation. However, they do still carry a small amount of positive attributes as a memory of what they once were in their whole food state. When the acquisition of whole, organic fruits and vegetables are beyond our budget or ability to purchase, we can ask in faith, with intention, that we be protected from any *negative resonance* included in our diets. This includes pesticides, herbicides, MSG in any and all forms, preservatives, additives, etc.

Remember though, God *knows* when we put our best foot forward and make the sacrifices necessary to eat well. When we do our best to eat well— it is acknowledged by God, and our faith will grow as a result. Eating well can mean a number of things to a number of different people. There is a variety of dietary advice and diet trends currently out. I would encourage you to ask for genes of **discernment in food consumption** to be turned on so you can be guided in what is true and untrue about these fads and trends.

When one is truly desirous for God's healing, He will require you to show *your* faith and diligence. He may encourage you to avoid certain foods and let go of previous food habits. When I was affected by Lyme symptoms, I felt very strongly, at one point, that I needed to stop consuming any and all grains, and eliminate animal products from my diet. I obeyed, and by adhering to these dietary guidelines, was able to function much better, and my pain was diminished. I also found that as I adhered to my dietary regime, I was not as fatigued as I would have been when consuming the foods I was impressed not to. I *really* desired to heal and to help others, so the motivation for me to comply was great.

I understand that it is difficult for many to adhere to dietary changes that are against the norm, and socially not accepted. But I promise as you diligently show your faith by your works, your efforts and ability to adhere to your inspired dietary changes will increase, and you can ask for more willpower to be given you. I cannot express to you how many of my patients have seen marked improvements in their health— emotional, physical and spiritual— *just* by changing their dietary intake to whole foods, and eliminating foods that don't possess enough light to help them heal.

Other factors that can affect our gene expression on a spiritual level (as well as physical) are chemical products. These include cleaning products, hair care products, colognes, perfumes, sanitizers, stains, paint, soaps, and more. Every product that has ever been produced will have a resonance to it. Some products are made in love, to improve quality of life, and are not created with components that are caustic or damaging to the environment. Others are produced with more deleterious chemicals, and contain multiple compounds that are synthetically made and toxic to the environment and our bodies.

These chemical residues and products, will have more of a negative resonance, as they are produced for ease, convenience, and profitability, instead of being more eco friendly to Mother Earth. Use discernment to know which products would be better for you to use in your home and with your family. One does not need to change everything all at once, but as you feel prompted to do so, make the changes required. Everything should be done in wisdom and order, and we should not run faster than we have strength.

Everything on this planet has resonance— it resonates from the emotions that were used to create it. Things created in fear or greed will bring more of the same, and things created in love bring more of the same. Remember this basic principle, and it will take you far on your healing journey. The more you make the appropriate changes, the more faith you will be demonstrating to be healed. If you cannot afford to change certain products in your home, you can pray in faith to have negative resonance removed from them. You will be blessed according to your faith. However, it is important to remember that God knows what you can and cannot change in your lifestyle. If we have the ability to change things for the better, we should do it.

During my health trial, I specifically remember using an ammonia-based cleaning solution in my bathrooms. Every time I used it, I felt worse, and headaches would ensue. After recognizing this pattern, I switched to a non-toxic solution and no longer had headaches when cleaning my home. Also switching my shower head to filter out chlorine from the water made a remarkable difference in my well being. Recognizing the small things you can do to show your faith and desire to be healed, and then making such changes, can bring about marked results. Pray to know what you should do regarding chemicals and products in your home.

Medical procedures also need to be discussed at this juncture, because they can promote, or inhibit, our ability to heal. When we look at the vastness of medical knowledge acquired to date— it is largely from scientific explanations performed by man. It is man's understanding of the human frame and how to care for it on a physical level. Yet, this knowledge, while it has its benefits, is self limiting. We are spiritual beings first, and as such, all things must be viewed with the spiritual lense for ultimate healing to occur. So much of medicine today is infused with fear. Fear that if we don't take an antibiotic we will get septic. Fear that we need to have a CT scan or an x ray because of a symptom. Then, when we may have a finding show up on that scan, the provider wants to run more tests and a potential trial of a medication. Thus, we can go down a path of depending upon medications and procedures to save us.

We become fearful because we don't know what is going on with our body, and then new symptoms develop. We search out a diagnosis to appease our mind, when in reality— it doesn't change the outcome. We go back to providers for more of the same, and often very little feedback is positive, encouraging, or uplifting. Worse still, when someone can't find a diagnosis, and nothing can be found, they continue to go to one specialist after another to find out "what is wrong," instead of focusing on the signals the body is giving them and attending to it directly. We neglect to ask God— the master Physician, what is going on with us, and what we should do to heal!

We forget about Him and forgo His power to heal us. When we take a medication, we are telling our body to manage symptoms. We are silencing the spirit, and we will never fully heal and be restored to full function until we break away from the dependency on man— and shift it to full dependency in God.

Medications can be helpful to someone who is in dire need, and does not yet have the gift of faith to be healed by God. But we should not forgo pursuit of complete healing and wholeness made possible by God. We are divine offspring— we possess the power to heal— and we should take full advantage of it! As a provider, I used to believe that certain medical interventions and medications were a blessing from God— that they were created to prevent and treat illness. But I have since realized they are produced by man, and are a telestial way of healing. It demonstrates the mercy of God. Indeed, He will meet us where we are at, according to our faith and desires to heal, but this modality does not directly address the root of the problem. As it does not fix the underlying problem, it takes away personal responsibility to get to the root of the symptom.

The belief that these modalities are the *best* way (instead of *a* way) to treat illness, has become an idea of mainstream acceptance in our society. It is a wile of the adversary that needs to be realized and understood before many can move forward to true healing. Surgical intervention may be necessary, and it is an amazing blessing to have such advancements at this time. Certain surgeries are designed to save lives! Others are designed to improve quality of life, or fix an acute problem of a greater magnitude. Some surgeries help repair disfigurement or physical defects. Others are designed to promote vanity and a fixation on personal appearance. Remember that every procedure, medical intervention, and medication has a *resonance* to it, and that resonance lingers within us.

Some things are created in greed, envy or lust— others are truly grown in love. Perceive with spiritual eyes to know whether you should incorporate such things into your being. See where your faith is, and what tools you need to gain the faith to be healed by God. If you feel a medication, at this time, is necessary, I encourage you to not feel bad about taking it. Explore all options available for healing, and then decide what is the next step to take. I would never judge anyone who has taken medications, as that too was part of my path to healing. But remember— you can pray over those medications so that the negative resonance can be removed, or that you will be protected from those influences.

Whatever you decide, never forgo progressing in faith toward the ultimate Healer so you can be completely healed! There are other supplements and supports that are derived from natural means and can support depression and other mood changes. Study these out as well, to see which of *all* the recommendations feels right, and proceed accordingly. We will **never** be able to receive the correct answer to our healing path if we do not explore ALL options and possibilities. Have an open mind and heart, be willing to shift towards new modalities that feel right, even if they are not conventional or mainstream. Cast out fear and doubt, and let faith and hope guide you.

Faith vs Doubt

Faith is atypical in its terminology. It is difficult to truly understand the scope and depth of the power of faith. It is a small word that bears with it great meaning. Faith is the means by which things unseen by man— are understood, by which the unexplainable— becomes explained, and clarity— rolls into perfection. Faith can have many different facets to it, and there are a variety of ways to develop faith. One can ask to have more faith, but as faith is a *very* broad topic, one will more readily receive the right kind of faith suited to their needs when they ask with specificity.

Faith in God is multiplanar. We can believe that God exists and sits on His throne above, and trust that He is aware of us. We can see Him as an all knowing being who stays above the earth and merely observes from that vantage point, or we can choose to develop that faith further. We can choose to exercise faith in God as a direct God to us, as a being who loves us unconditionally and completely, and is very aware of our needs and wants. We can view Him thus, as in the trenches, walking the earth, observing the details of His children. This faith allows us to feel more connected to Him and His love. Even further, we can choose to view Him as a part of US— literally, that we are intimately and completely connected to Him as His child, that He is walking beside us *always*, and we are never separate from Him. When we can reach this realization, a growing ability to access His power and learn of His ways occurs.

Faith can grow from a lesser understanding and belief until it becomes a knowing, an absolute truth residing in the mind and heart of the individual. It is a beautiful process, as if a rose is unfolding in view, accepting the gifts of the sun, rain, and air to sustain it. Building this type of faith takes work and endurance and determination. It requires that we be willing to **not** accept the acceptable in society, that we reject the mistruths and philosophies of man, and strive to find God's truth in all things— in every way and form. It creates a willingness to submit to His will in all things, trust in His timetable, and be open to change. As we do this, faith grows within us, and it leads us to hope for those things that are not seen. We can therefore hope that we will one day be healed, or possess the power to heal.

Like faith, hope in healing also can grow. We can hope that one day we will be healed, and wait patiently on the Lord, making little or no effort to change our lifestyle. This is a more passive exercise of hope. A greater exercise in hope is to do EVERYTHING you feel is correct to unlock more faith and hope in healing. This can motivate one to seek out God's truth and information regarding their symptoms and illness, apply nutritional and supplemental advice that is sound and correct, and continue *enduring* till the end of the trial of health.

Enduring to the end means holding true to the promptings and answers you have received from God and not vacillate. Period. It means not throwing in the towel when you don't see immediate results, or jumping from one provider to the next to get another opinion unless you feel prompted to by the spirit. If you have received your answer from God that you should adhere to a particular regime, stick with it! It may need alteration and that is when you can ask Him if there is something more to be done.

I would encourage you not to step off your path to healing when there are some hiccups along the way. We are meant to experience adversity, we are meant to have difficulty. It is often a rollercoaster ride when we set the intention to heal according to God's will. Often we forgo the "quick fix" promised by society and decide to traverse through unchartered territory. The path may, at times, feel lonely and dark, as those around us do not understand or know how to help us. We may be ridiculed by others, who believe we are doing everything wrong. God is aware of this, and we are never left alone, even if we feel such. He is always sending angels, light, and love, as we are open to *receive* it.

This path to healing is not an easy one— it isn't meant to be. How are we to expect great growth and understanding into the mysteries of God without a personally tailored trial? How can we more fully develop empathy and love for others who are struggling, if we don't pass through struggles of our own? Indeed, life is not always easy, it was never designed to be such. This realization is not new, but it is often an unwelcome concept. However, when we are hit with a really difficult emotional, physical or spiritual trial— we have the agency to choose how to move through it. We can decide to be miserable, or angry and frustrated, or we can choose to look upward and outward.

When we choose to ask God for help through this trial, we can literally receive greater insight and understanding into the reasons behind the trial, and what is to be learned. We can ask for specific genes to be manifest (hope, faith, charity) that will strengthen us and uplift us when the times are not just tough, but seemingly insurmountable. We can choose to serve others in our even limited capacity, and demonstrate faith to lift others amidst our own difficulties. Or we can do the opposite. We can choose to linger in solitude and misery, and look at others who have it "easy" in disgust. We can choose to be angry for the hand we have been dealt and decide that we no longer will communicate with God.

This behavior not only promotes the continuation of illness, but it may cut off other avenues of positive reinforcement we so desperately need! Often friends and family members will initially be supportive and helpful when we enter a trial of health. But if we choose bitterness and negativity, those resources will eventually be dried up and desertion may occur. I have met some dear people who are struggling deeply, but have become enveloped in a dark cloud of anger, and thus are not progressing in upward movement to God. They will never be able to heal in this manner, and thus continue down a path of indecision, discomfort, and doubt.

You are validated to feel frustration or discouragement at times. This is natural, and part of the process of mourning during illness. But I would encourage you not to linger long there— ask to be lifted above those negative emotions. Asking forgiveness from our negative attitudes or emotions, opens the door to healing, and a softening of our hearts. Doing this daily puts you in direct contact with the Holy Spirit, so you can be guided, directed, and strengthened in your decisions, thoughts, and actions.

Sometimes, the internal negativity grows so great that you literally cannot find a well of light and hope within you. If this is the case, seek out ways to bring light into your being, through uplifting music, meditation, sunshine, words of affirmation, scriptures, inspired messages and quotes, healthy foods, and the right supplements. These can all infuse you with faith and hope and shift your mindset to the positive. At times of dark depression, medication may need to be prescribed. You will be the judge of that. But always think of the end goal— to gain complete resolution of all symptoms through Christ, the Master Healer.

Faith in God is imperative to heal. However, there cannot be full resolution of symptoms unless you have faith in yourself! Do you truly and fully believe that you can heal or be healed? Do you trust your intuition and the guidance you receive through the Spirit? If you answered "no" to either of these questions, do not be alarmed! Faith in oneself is a concept that is understood with time. In order to receive faith in ourselves, we must ask for it first.

Specifically pray and ask that genes of faith in yourself be turned on, as well as genes of trust in yourself. Ask for genes of doubt or disbelief in your abilities be silenced and the triggers removed. It is possible that not every doubt or disbelief will be silenced by this process— indeed we have to experience opposition! But you will find that you have more confidence, and you'll be able to trust in yourself with greater ease by performing these exercises.

We can learn to trust ourselves as we follow God's counsel and personal impressions of the spirit. It is important to note, however, that we will *only* receive impressions based on the knowledge we have gained. If we have not looked at *all* avenues and paths to healing, we may be missing a vital piece of information that could prove to our advantage, and ultimately guide us to complete health. Intuition and insight are only based on the knowledge and understanding of the individual. We will not receive inspiration, out of the blue, for ourselves, or someone else, regarding some new technique or modality, if we never have taken the time to explore it.

When I became very ill, I was fortunate to receive the right information regarding my illness. It was a missing piece of information I needed to put the complete puzzle of health together. That missing piece came from a source that I would not have normally considered, but I took it to the Lord and asked in faith. After receiving my confirmed answer, I proceeded forth and never looked back. You will be guided and directed to what *you* need to do to heal, provided you keep an open mind and heart, and ask in faith for God to direct you to the truth. Actively search out *all* modalities of healing to encounter the one (or many) that feel right for you. Seek out the truth behind your illness, so you can align to the correct treatment plan for you, and proceed forward in faith.

Serving others brings feelings of self-worth, and activates more faith in yourself. I would encourage you to consider its incorporation on your path to healing. It can be a simple phone call or letter to someone in need, or a completely new idea! Serving others when you are feeling your worst, literally accelerates and enhances the healing process. As you proceed forth in service, with a positive attitude and true desire to help others, you will find less discomfort with time. You will be infused with more faith and optimism, despite your current circumstances and feel more confident in your ability to heal.

If faith is the first principle to healing, then what are the effects of doubt? Doubt is in direct opposition to faith. When we doubt, we are pulled down into the darkness of negativity. We start to question everything— we become unsure of our progress, or our path to healing. We begin to distrust in the things we once felt were right and true. It's also important to remember—fear is the fuel to doubt.

How often do you leave your healthcare provider's office feeling joyful and uplifted? If the answer is rarely or never, I would encourage you to find a provider that will cheer you on in your decisions and endeavors to heal, that will not belittle you or ridicule you, or make you feel inferior. Each of us possess the ability to heal our very frames, and each of us can be guided in how to do so. Healing is the responsibility of the *person*— not the physician, or provider, or other healer. Remember this!

No power on earth (medical procedure, physician, specialist, etc.) can heal you. Only God's power, through your incredible faith, can heal you. Period. When you've been sick with the flu before, or had a surgical intervention and you healed— it was done by the Spirit, which organized and healed the physical body. Indeed, we can take in certain foods and supports to enhance our ability to heal, but the Spirit is the foundation of healing.

Spiritual genes affect immune function on a *physical* level. Without the spiritual influence, we would not be able to recover and heal, and would have been long ago deceased on this planet. Without the spiritual DNA, there would be no life— no procreation, no healing, no progression. When thoughts of doubt start to creep into your mind, quickly ask God for thoughts of optimism and hope! You can ask for positive images to fill your mind, or turn on a meditation that is uplifting to you. Sing a positive song, write an inspired mantra and use it over and over when you feel the raindrops of doubt fall upon you. In so doing, you are putting up an umbrella of faith and hope, and can be protected from doubt.

The more you turn to optimism— the more optimism will grow. Like seeds in a harvest— you will reap what you sow. Strive to sow seeds of hope and goodwill towards others— and your garden will be replete with fragrant flowers to cheer you up on dreary days. And let us not forget— you can let the sunshine of faith flow through you to nourish these seeds as they grow within you. If we do not doubt, we will receive the greatest bounty of faith to be healed!

> *"And whosoever shall believe in my name, doubting **nothing**, unto him will I confirm all my words, even unto the ends of the earth."*
> Mormon 9:25

He has promised the very faithful, power to be healed in this life. Shall we not take Him up on the offer?

> *"And again, it shall come to pass that he who hath faith in me to be healed, and is not appointed unto death, shall be healed."*
> D&C 42:48

Notice it doesn't say "maybe" be healed. For those who grow and develop a powerful faith in our Heavenly Father through their *exact* obedience, He is bound by His word to heal them in *this* life— if they are not appointed to death. The adversary's bounds are set, and he cannot take our life from us. We have our time appointed to return home. Yet, he can definitely make our lives miserable if we allow it. Let us choose to lift one another, and in so doing, lift ourselves. This way, we are able to cast out doubt and fear, and grow in faith and hope.

I testify the power of service is real! As I struggled throughout my life with poor self-esteem, lack of confidence, depression, anxiety, and more, I found myself drawn to service. At a young age, I recognized the power of service to lift others and it helped me feel better as well. Service was the saving grace that brought me joy, peace, and strength amid the struggles and vicissitudes of life. I saw those around me as my brothers and sisters, and serving was a way to show gratitude and love to God. Through this gift of service, He has blessed me immensely to reject the adversary and the negativity in the world today— and He can do the same for you.

C H A P T E R 5

Turning to Light

When we return to God, it would be wonderful to be free of any negative emotion. Throughout history, sin has been given a negative connotation that is derived from beliefs that God is a being to be feared, and separate from. This is a falsehood, and is a doctrine designed by the adversary to divide man from God. In its essence, sin is merely anything that makes us feel separation from God.

For some people, they allow themselves to be overburdened with "sins," or little acts and misgivings, that are quite trivial in nature. This creates a large chasm between them and God, and they don't believe they can reach out for His goodness. Others may *not* view their deeds and misgivings of a larger nature as a sin, and may neglect to ask forgiveness so that they may be filled with the Holy Spirit. This can lead them down a path of spiritual apathy, becoming numb to emotions of guilt and sorrow, and altogether foregoing God's presence in their lives. God is aware of each of us and our individual needs for repentance.

Sometimes we are too hard on ourselves, and view every little mistake as a great stumbling block into His presence. This is again a tool of the adversary. God is always standing with His arms outstretched, ready to envelop us in His love. We are the ones who feel unjustified before Him. He loves us as we do our best and try to change bad habits. All too often, when we ask forgiveness of God for a "sin" or a deed that separates us from Him, we neglect to forgive ourselves! If we don't forgive ourselves, we cannot move forward. The Lord forgives and forgets our sins when we truly repent— shall not we?

"Behold, he who has repented of his sins, the same is
forgiven, and I, the Lord, remember them no more."
D&C 58:42

In order to receive miracles of healing, we need to be prepared to see ourselves as perfect before Him. This means clean every whit, free of any and all sins through our repentance and faith. We have to be accepting of this reality, or healing cannot occur. When we repent, the Holy Spirit can reside within us, and literally change the manifestation of our desires, wants, and wishes. We can experience a mighty change in our hearts, where we "no longer desire to do evil, but wish to do good continually." (Mosiah 5:2)

This change can occur rapidly when we, in humility, come to the Lord, and ask Him to take our burdens and challenges. We must be willing to let go of control and hand everything over to Him. Removing all the lies and negativity of the adversary from our hearts, we can place them on the sacrificial altar. Once there, we can watch them disappear, and replace them with the truth of who we really are, and the love God has for us.

At times, we may need to ask what it is that we need to repent of, in order to move forward. Sometimes, it may be as simple as unbelief, or being blind in our hearts— unable to see the truth that is right in front of us. Often, it may be impatience, time wasting, or pride.

Remember that sin is anything that separates you from God. This can be due to your own *perception* that you have gone against God's will— one of the adversary's tactics, making you think you aren't good enough. It's important to remember, a true misdeed that requires repentance, will often demonstrate itself as a prompting of the Spirit, and you will know in your conscience.

The closer you are to the Spirit, the more you will recognize the things for which you need to ask forgiveness. And the more you are repentant and pure before the Lord, and *accept* your own offering of forgiveness, you will often find that the things you once thought were mountains of sin, are truly smaller molehills!

As you align to God, and find His truth in all things, you may be led to an organized religion wherein His complete truth is found. Do not fear this step. Making covenants, or promises with God— as did Abraham— strengthens our resolve to follow Him, and gives us an additional power to overcome this world. It opens up the spiritual DNA to more light, and unlocks more spiritual gifts! It also allows us to "bind" the Lord by His word, as we follow our part of the agreement. Participating in the ordinances of the gospel, and keeping covenants made with Christ, are an essential part of returning home to our Heavenly Parents.

Recognize, however, that any religion which depicts a punishing God, who likes to hurt or berate His children, is *not* His truth. Know this, and prevent the pitfall of feeling more separated from God by this belief. God is full of patience, long suffering, and love unfeigned. He is always available to attend to your needs, and the desires of your heart— any time of day, and any way you feel the need to communicate with Him in light. If you do not feel He is listening, or you do not see immediate results of your communication with Him, it may be because you are imposing your will on His. You are asking for what you *want*, instead of what God knows you *need*.

Sometimes you may not receive the answer because there is some information you need to learn, or seek out first, in order to build up your knowledge and understanding, and thus receive your answer. So often, I would pray, wanting the answer for a patient's condition, and nothing would come. I literally wanted the heavens to open and receive *all* light and knowledge on a topic without working to receive it! God doesn't work this way— He requires us to acquire knowledge to build upon, and then He inspires us along the way. These are important things to consider in prayer.

As we submit to His will, and are willing to *wait* according to His timetable, and continue learning, we will be blessed. Waiting on His timetable for healing is *not* sedentary— it means you are going to do your best to demonstrate your faith by action. These actions include, serving others, studying His words, pondering His power, and finding out the truest desires of your heart as you turn to Him. It means you will be willing to work to fill your body with light from the foods and supplements you may be guided to, and be willing to give up certain habits, foods, or medications, when you feel prompted to do so. Everyone will have a different way to manifest their faith, and we all will have certain limitations. But He will know whether you are striving to do your best and He will love you for your efforts.

As you are prompted by the Spirit to ask forgiveness of any misdeeds or errors that are preventing you from accessing His help to heal, remember that sometimes this process takes time. There may be things required at your hand to fully bring restitution of the situation. If you have hurt others by your actions, you will be asked to do your best to repair those relationships and ask forgiveness of those whom you have affected. If you stole something, you will be asked to replace it, and be honest from here on out in your dealings with others. If you have been critical of others, you must completely *cease* to criticize them, and ask forgiveness of them and God.

If you have followed the promptings of the Spirit, and done all that was required for true forgiveness to be granted, remember the *last* step is to forgive yourself fully, completely, and forever. This means not dwelling on the past, and not allowing the mistakes of twenty years ago take up residence in your mind and heart. It means letting it go, releasing it to the Lord, and allowing Him to take the burden away from you.

All too often, we ask for forgiveness and we picture ourselves giving the burden to God, and yet the next day, we may turn around and take it back, or engage in the same negative behavior. This is not full repentance. It is still a step in the right direction, if you are actively trying to give up a bad habit or a negative behavior that prevents you from accessing God's power to heal you. He will know if you are asking forgiveness with a sincere desire to change and turn toward Him, or if it is just a "vain repetition," or going through the motions to appease others in your life, or pretend to be more righteous than you truly are.

Make sure that when you ask forgiveness, you are truly, sincerely, wanting to change. The stronger your will and desire to make such changes in your life, the more God will empower you from above with the ability to overcome *any* and all negative desires, appetites or passions. This includes addictions. Addictions are a great tool of the adversary designed to keep us in a holding pattern wherein there is no progression. It promotes a cycle of guilt, and then we engage in the same behavior, because of the darkness we feel. It becomes a temporary relief, and then down we go again.

Addictions may be difficult to overcome, but as you strive to make your will God's will— you can overcome any and all trials. This is a promise, and the more you cling to Him and ask for His help to overcome in faith, and covenant with Him, the more power will be granted unto you to do so. You will receive more guidance on how this is to be done, and what you can do to fill your life with goodness, so as to take away the constant stream of addictive thoughts and desires.

This is yet another miracle on its own— overcoming addictions as you come to God fully, and with real intent! It is part of the healing process, and will be granted unto you as you pursue this journey to healing by God's power. If you need additional support, you can ask God to turn off genes of regret, and then ask for genes of oneness and wholeness in God, to be turned on. Make sure all genes of faith are turned on, and if you have specific fears regarding your addiction— triggers that set you off, then ask specifically for the gene of that particular fear to be silenced, and the trigger removed.

Ask also, for genes of fortitude, wisdom, humility, power to overcome and genes of sanctity to be turned on. Anytime you are triggered, and it sends you into cravings— stop and recognize the trigger. Then ask for that trigger to be removed, and to silence any negative emotions associated with that trigger. Focus on others and serve, serve, serve! If this is done in full faith— overcoming addictions will become much easier than has historically been done.

Remember, you are a child of God— and as such, you can have access through the Holy Spirit to overcome *anything*. It is in your DNA— it is who you truly are. Sometimes you must continue to ask for silencing of those genes of fear, and removal of triggers, as it is a pattern which must be broken over time. Continue to do your best and your efforts will be magnified! You will see progression more quickly when you seek help from above.

We must also recognize the importance of forgiving others of their mistakes. Often, we hold onto hurt feelings or disappointment regarding another's decisions or actions. This does not injure the individual to whom we have these emotions— but it does prevent us from progressing. No one is perfect in this life, indeed each of us will error. That is why Christ's sacrifice was necessary, so we could remove the residues of indiscretion from our chapters. Is it not amazing, that Christ who suffered for everyone, and has all power to withhold forgiveness as a result, chooses to forgive us daily? Despite the pain and suffering He went through, He would do it all over again for *just you*, because of His deep and abiding love for you.

The Savior wants us to follow His example and forgive others. He has all power to make things right in the end, and we can trust Him in His promises. We may not see full resolution to a discordant situation in *this* life due to agency of others, but we can know that everything will be made whole and complete in the next. Trusting this, we can move forward and look towards the great day of happiness when all tears will be wiped away and all sorrow forgotten. Yet, in this life, we must choose to forgive.

> *"I will forgive whom I will forgive, but of you*
> *it is required to forgive all men."*
> D&C 64:10

Why are we encouraged, even commanded to forgive? Because God knows what it will do to our heart and soul if we don't! We will continue to transcribe our DNA in anger, frustration, and hurt— it will introduce darkness into our soul. Forgiveness brings light, a brilliant light that is unlike any other. This is because the light of Christ is essential to forgiving another, and ourselves. We must become like Him in order to forgive, and therefore, the greatest frequency of light is incorporated into our being as we do so. If we do not forgive, we will be prone to the darkness of disease at some point in our lives. To those who forgive, they receive promised blessings of peace and joy in this life. They are filled with hope and can move forward and progress in light.

It starts with faith that God can help change your heart. Pray for His help to let go of the hurt and anger. With time, your heart will soften, and eventually, you will be free from the negative emotions you have wrestled with for so long. When I have forgiven others, I envision myself handing all that dark negativity up to Christ, and it disappears in a flume of light. Sometimes incorporating visualization such as this can also help you let go of the emotions stifling your progress. Asking for genes of forgiveness and redemption to be opened for transcription will also aid this process, as it is done in faith. You can also ask that genes of emotional remembrance from that negative experience be silenced, and any triggers removed when you have fully processed the situation and forgiven the offender(s).

As we repent, or ask forgiveness of any wrongdoing, we are filled with more light, and the love of God, as we recognize His power to forgive and forget. We are more willing to undergo even further transformation toward Him, and to become more like Him— even if it means going against the cultural and social norms of our day. When we achieve forgiveness, we literally are turning our hearts and minds to God. We are asking Him to change us in a real way, in not only a spiritual state, but a physical one. The spiritual DNA actually changes form and function.

When we *receive* forgiveness, genes of gratitude, hope, joy, peace, and faith in ourselves, are opened and transcribed. We feel lighter—no longer weighed down, and we may feel physically stronger as well. This is because our spirit is overcoming the selfish desires of the natural man, or ego; and thus, the power of our spirit over our body is made manifest. You are divine, you have always existed— and you will always be blessed when you make correct choices in alignment to God.

In the DNA, there are the genes of mortality. They will always be with us, and it is a beautiful reminder of the physical life we live here on the earth. Some of these genes help us to proceed forward in light, and learn the lessons of God. Others are inhibitory and prevent progression in the spiritual sense (negative emotions and experiences in our chapters). Both types of genes, or "chapters," are necessary for our growth, and cannot be discounted. We have to experience the evil to know the good and appreciate the pureness and joy of life when it is found. We have to know the struggle of sorrow and feeling separation from God, and we have to understand spiritual, emotional, and physical pain. All of these emotions and experiences are situated within the DNA and are transcribed into the sinews of our very souls.

This process of communication from physical to the spiritual begins with the heart and mind. In scripture, there are countless verses that discuss turning hearts to God. When we focus on turning to God, when we communicate with Him through our minds *and* our hearts, prayer becomes substantially more powerful. The most meaningful prayers I have ever spoken were when I knelt before my Creator in gratitude and wonder, expressing the deepest reverence and respect for His power, and thanking Him for all that I have been given. These prayers were often said in my darkest, most difficult trials. Prayers of gratitude are powerful!

It is important to ask for His help in our lives, but often it is joyful to just thank Him for all we are, all we've been, and all we will be, through Christ. We begin to recognize all our innumerable blessings, and therefore increase in love towards Him, from whence all blessings flow. Recited prayers can hold meaning and have purpose, but truly to express the desires of your heart— these prayers are supernal indeed.

As we embrace this type of prayer, we may find we are sharing things with Him that we thought were long buried deep, or already dealt with, or not important. God is our Father, and He wants us to talk with Him! He wants to hear our joys and triumphs, and our struggles and sorrows. He wants to succor us in every point of this mortal journey, but we must let Him in. He will not force His way into our hearts— we must come to Him. It is our personal agency at play— we make the choice to approach Him and knock.

"Ask, and it shall be given you; seek, and ye shall find; knock, and it shall be opened unto you: For every one that asketh receiveth; and he that seeketh findeth; and to him that knocketh it shall be opened."
Matthew 7:7-8

The desires of our heart need to be in alignment with God. When the heart is in alignment to God, our mind is as well. All your actions, desires, and thoughts, will be transcribed into the DNA in love, light, and trust— if your eye is single to God. The body will become filled with light, and darkness will be cast out. The genes, or experiences and traits that were once so cumbersome to us— the lessons you are given over and over to learn, will then be conquered, and you will find that you see others differently, including yourself.

You will see the beauty of every one of God's children, even if they are making choices that seem detrimental to their progression. You will feel love and acceptance of who they are and where they are at— and this includes yourself! You will see the earth differently, in her splendor and majesty, and have a desire to connect with and care for her. During the continual process of turning to God, you literally turn on more and more of the positive genes for self-realization and manifestation in creating, and silence the genes of self-doubt, judgement, anger, and selfishness.

The desires of your heart can and *will* change as you make an effort to fill your life with love. Serving others despite difficulty, seeking out God's truth from the best books and sources, learning to feel Him and receive guidance of the Spirit, and sincere and powerful prayer, make this possible. This is a process that starts with faith— or the desire to believe it can be so. And as you plant the seed of faith in your heart, and nourish it with hope, trust, and love— it will grow and blossom until your very being emanates the love of God for everything around you. You will have patience and understanding unlike you've ever experienced, and you will make inspired decisions regarding your life's path. You will desire to serve God with all you've been given, and seek to do His will in all things.

When your heart is full of His love— your mind will constantly be thinking of Him, and how you can bring His love to others— you will echo the words of eternity. His power will be within you, and you will watch your physical ailments improving day by day, here a little and there a little, until you **no longer experience them.** Turning the DNA towards God means you will open up to Him and be vulnerable, and ask His forgiveness, and His guidance for you. It means you are willing to accept His will and timeline for your healing, and the miracle of restoration to health.

You demonstrate the desires of your heart everyday by what you desire to do, how you think and act, and where you spend your time. Ask yourself this personal question— truly, where is my heart? What do I spend my time doing? What could I sacrifice more to show complete faith and devotion to God? One does not need to be a Bible scholar, or study scriptures for hours on end! But one could cut out substantial time from social media, television shows, and other sources that do not uplift, and focus more on studying His words, serving others, meditating, or pondering the deeper meaning of life.

Words are powerful! Did you know as we study scriptures and God's words, it provides us with a greater power to shift the DNA in the right direction? Literally, as we read God's words, the emotions of love, gratitude, and hope we feel in our hearts by that process, upregulate gene transcription and translation! We turn on more genes of light, and silence more genes of darkness (or negativity or illness). Similarly, if we speak or read things that are not full of charity and kindness, we are allowing ourselves to be acted upon by the adversary— and we will shift away from the DNA of Godliness, and hold less power to heal.

Words have the power to unlock the door to complete resolution of symptoms, or to project you down a prolonged path of suffering and regret. Words you speak tell others what you are thinking and feeling— including your very DNA! God's words, when obtained in their perfect form, are designed to speak to your soul— to remind you of your divinity and who you truly are. They are on the earth today to provide a connection from heaven to earth, to call us to repentance, to purify us, and allow His light and love to flow freely into our hearts and souls.

Words hold deeper meaning, and multiple definitions of words can be evaluated and measured. As you study God's words, look for the similarities and differences of the multiple meanings one word can have. In so doing, you will unlock even more power of gene transcription, and obtain more diversity in gene expression towards light and oneness. Seek out the words of God in their purest form, free from the philosophies of man, or altered by limited translation. The purer you can find God's words, the more powerful gene transcription and translation will become.

Another powerful exercise is to write down your feelings and beliefs in God— expressing your love to Him, your confidence in His power to heal you, and your willingness to come to Him and learn of Him. Writing down inspired words such as these also turns on transcription of the DNA, and provides you with more light, more expression of the positive genes and emotions, and will help diminish the darkness (or negativity, or disease). The first portion of the Bible indicates that in the beginning, there was the Word. Jesus Christ is the Word— and the power of the Word (or words) are great.

*"In the beginning was the Word, and the Word
was with God, and the Word was God."*
John 1:1

Christ has experienced every one of our sorrows, misgivings, errors, sicknesses, and tribulations. He transcribed the spiritual DNA on our behalf in Gethsemane. We cannot imagine the intense suffering and pain it caused Him to experience such things. He transcribed our challenging "words" one by one, making this sacrifice a real and personal one for each individual. As such, He is the perfect editor and coauthor, and his vocabulary bank is *endless*. He is able to eliminate any negative wording, and replace it with positive phrases, as we turn to Him. Everything in the Universe is created with words—and His words are endless and powerful. We can incorporate His words into our ladder of life by following His example, and asking for His help when we make mistakes.

Another way to incorporate the power of words is through music. Songs which sing praises unto God allow us to demonstrate our devotion to Him, and express gratitude and love for His creations. We are heard by God and the angels when we sing, and it becomes a sweet melody to their ears, even if we lack the talent of perfect pitch. As we sing praises to God, the words hold deeper resonance and power as they are coupled with music. The vibratory sensation of a word put to song is more powerful than the word alone, and can enhance and speed up the process of healing. It increases our energy frequency, and diminishes the lower frequencies of doubt, depression, or darkness.

Make good selective choices about the music you allow in your space when you are striving to heal. Uplifting hymns or choral music can fill you with more love and light, especially when you are down or depressed. When I was in the lowest, darkest parts of my struggle with Lyme symptoms, I had music, scriptures, or talks by inspired men and women, playing ALL day. Their words helped lift me and gave me light, faith, and hope to get me through those extremely difficult times. Music, alone, can also lift us, and shift us, when it is positive in tempo, rhythm, and motion.

As you listen to music, check in with how you are feeling, and ask yourself— is this lifting me up, or pulling me down? This exercise will help you decipher what music choices are good for you. The day after I was completely healed by God, I turned on some hymns— and "Come Thou Fount" played over three times in a row on my streaming device! I feel it is a message that this particular song holds great power to heal the human frame, and would encourage you to incorporate listening to it or singing it daily.

I have a dear friend who struggled with knee pain for years. She was inspired to write a song of love for her knee and sing to it daily! Interestingly enough, her pain diminished as she incorporated this exercise. Words hold power to heal, and selective words, directed in love to your body, will literally accelerate the healing process. When I was chronically ill, I prayed everyday in gratitude for my body. I expressed my amazement and wonder at its intricacies, and how it was doing such a great job at fighting off the viral infections. I asked specifically that my white blood cells and other immunoglobulins (immune system components) would function properly, and be activated appropriately. The more specific you can be with your words in prayers of faith, the more specifically God can bless you. The more you express love and appreciation for your soul, the more it will accelerate your healing.

You are collectively a sum of expressions, experiences, words, and emotions. These are all stored in our DNA and make us who we are. We have the power and ability to align ourselves to God and access His power to heal. We do this through altering our emotional reactions to experiences, by the words we choose to use, what we choose to read or hear, what we think or do, and ultimately— who we truly want to become. The desire of our heart must be to be in alignment with God in all things. The faith to believe it will happen is what brings our progression toward Him, as we demonstrate our faith through our actions. When we can align our heart's desire to

His, personal improvement is propelled forward at an expedited pace, and is far easier than trying to do so from a "things to work on" list. And we experience expedited healing too!

Trust

*"Trust in the Lord with all thine heart; and lean
not unto thine own understanding. In all thy ways
acknowledge him, and he shall direct thy paths."*
Proverbs 3:5-6

How can we trust completely in God? One cannot trust God unless they know Him. We can know *of* Him by reading scriptures that discuss His qualities and characteristics, but to truly *know* Him, we must come to Him in a real and sincere way. We do this by demonstrating faith and belief in Him through our thoughts, our actions, and our willingness to serve our fellow man. We learn to see— with the eye of faith, all that He has created and cared for, and even is continuing to create. We consider the cosmos of the universe in their expansion before us, and His greatness and glory that surrounds our human frames. We recognize that we are part of Him, as His creation, and we have the exact same potential to be like Him.

Let me repeat that— we have the **exact same potential** to become like God! This is an eternal truth. The more we familiarize ourselves with this doctrine of becoming like God, the more readily our spirit will be open to receiving gifts from above, which will align us to God. We are created in His own likeness and image. He is a personage, just as we are— our loving Father in Heaven.

*"So God created man in his own image, in the image of God
created he him; male and female created he them."*
Genesis 1:27

How can a man trust in someone whom he has never met? We must meet with God *daily* in our prayers— in our supplication to Him, from the depths of our hearts. Meditation, study, and pondering of who He is, also will help us understand His will more fully for us. I remember once asking Him what He feels like, and the image of a huge, massive mountain came to my mind, one whose peak was endless. A stormy sea being calmed, passed through my mind, and I felt this enormous, peaceful power that was solid and unchanging. It helped me identify with Him more in a beautiful way.

We can ask God what He looks like, and allow Him to paint a picture in our mind's eye. We can ask Him what His love for us feels like, what He desires for us, and ultimately— what our potential is as His child. When we can understand even the smallest bit of who God truly is, it helps us to recognize who we truly are in a powerful way. The more we reach up to God, and ask questions with fervor, the more He will be willing to give us the answers.

As we are open to receiving these answers— receiving often means *applying* the new knowledge to our lives, the more knowledge He will give us. The more we converse with Him, the more we understand and know God. The more we know and understand God, the more we will know and understand ourselves. And when we reach a level of such familiarity— we will trust Him implicitly. This means that we will not be swayed by the beliefs of men— we will be willing to stand as a light amidst the darkness of doubt. We will be able to overcome insurmountable trials and tribulations, because we will know that He is on our side. We will be able to unlock the power within our soul to continue going, to press on…and eventually, to completely heal!

We are not a sole entity, but connected to a greater knowing and understanding, which is our Heavenly Father. We are children of the most powerful force in the Universe— indeed, God! Is that not awe-inspiring? Does it not send chills down your spine, and light you as a flame to your very core? You are divine! You were chosen at *this* time and to be in *this* place for a specific purpose. He wants you to know you are loved, beyond measure. You are infinite, and always will be His. He wants you to trust Him in all things— He wants you to be made whole.

Trusting Him in all things may mean forgoing health recommendations from a friend, family member, or other individuals, despite their logic. It may mean trying a whole new way to heal, incorporating modalities that you've never explored or felt drawn to before. Indeed, it often will mean throwing the man-made manual to a "healthy and happy life" out the window, and starting over with the Healer himself. It often means patience, temperance, long suffering, and a willingness to submit to His timing for the resolution of things— while you seek out His truth, and His answers to help you manage the situation better.

Trusting in God means not lending yourself to other beliefs or "systematic" therapies— it means going to the source of all that is good and true, and making sense of His recommendations for you. Thinking outside the box is a huge endeavor, but it is often what God requires us to do in order to develop this magnitude of faith and trust. He is not an "in the box" thinker, by the way! He often requires us to have adaptable thoughts and be open to shifting them, applying them in a new way, or receiving a new concept into an already-integrated belief system. Fluidity is the word that comes to mind— we need to be willing to trust Him in His fluidity or grace, shifting our thought patterns as He desires us to. This is done from a lower level of understanding to reach a higher level of understanding.

Remember, all of this is done of our own will! He never will take agency away. But those who exercise their agency fully and without restraint, towards Him and His light, will be infinitely blessed. I remember when I was learning about chemistry, biology, and the foundational principles in science— these were more concrete ideas. Then I moved into the areas of medicine, which still required concrete science and knowledge, but also a development of "common sense" in the application of that knowledge. Then I was pushed into a new way of thinking, bridging from medication prescriptions, into herbal therapies and functional medicine— a more intuitive way.

Finally, I was encouraged to make yet another transition from this way of practicing into a completely new way of healing through spiritual epigenetics! If I had not allowed myself to be open to new things, and built my knowledge and understanding line upon line, precept on precept, I would not have been granted access to some of the most beautiful and wonderful concepts that only God can teach. As these processes are unknown to man, it would have been impossible to obtain them through study and application at a temporal university.

As God is in the universe— should we not attend His university? Often to gain this appreciation and understanding, we have to start at the basics, or what man *can* know and explain. From there, we can take what is needed to build our knowledge base further, and continue upward, discarding mistruths, or false beliefs of man, as we ascribe to God's truth in all things. Similar to my journey and education, each of us can attain knowledge of truth in all things, as we use discernment in our research and study.

If you feel confusion in this process, take a moment to pause, and reflect, and ask. Wait for further answers to come. Sometimes the phrase "Be still and know that I am God" will come to you, indicating it is a moment of reflection and waiting patiently for Him. He often will not give you knowledge continually, but allow you time to develop new skills and integrate the new information He has given you. As you work to incorporate new information into your life, God will bless you for it. More light and knowledge from above will come, and you will find yourself receiving an increasing amount of inspiring information. But to obtain this, we must trust God implicitly.

When you trust God implicitly, what happens? You will often find that making decisions become easier as you consult with Him. You will find that your path of research and study into healing modalities becomes streamlined and directed by Him. You will be led to the truth of what is required for you to fully heal, instead of wading through mountains of mistruths, or partial truths in health. In essence, you will reduce the amount of time you have been struggling with illness, because you will not be led to paths that bring only partial restoration to health.

You will also trust *yourself*, in a real and beautiful way. This self-confidence blossoms, and you will know and understand who you are, and thus stand in *your* truth— in all things. You will feel powerful and motivated, respectful of yourself and others, and you will be filled with love. You will not fear. Let me repeat that— **you will not fear**. When you trust God implicitly, there is no room for fear to abide. Your thoughts are one with Him— there is no doubt, no regret and no worry. You know He will take care of you and guide you, wherever you go and whatever you feel you should do.

When you trust in God implicitly, there will be appropriate concern for the calamities of our day, but a deep and abiding peace in knowing that you are where you need to be. There is no worry for the outcome and aftermath of material destruction, because you know that you are eternal and you are God's beloved child. You know without a doubt, He will take care of you and be with you always. This trust begins with faith in Him, and proceeds from there, as you earnestly seek His will and learn of Him, and reject the falsehoods of this world. It is a beautiful reciprocation between you and God, wherein more love and trust is created and becomes boundless.

If you have experienced broken trust in a relationship, it may be difficult to express trust in God. If this has happened to you, do not lose hope! If you have a desire, or wish you could develop this trust in God, that is the place to start. There are specific genes that can be accessed to help you gain trust in Him. First, ask that all genes of faith in God, and in yourself, be turned on. If you still remember, and are triggered by the situation of broken trust, ask God if you can silence the negative emotions tied to that memory (or memories) and remove the triggers. Ask for genes of hope in restoration to be turned on, as well as love of God, love of self, and love of fellowman. Ask for genes of remembrance of divinity and oneness to be turned on. Then ask for genes of reciprocity, recognition, and light to be open for transcription.

You are welcome to ask for this multiple times— even daily. You will feel things shifting as you ask with your heart and mind. More hope and trust will emerge from you, and you will find an ability to confide in God again. If you have been angry with God, and felt that He was not there for you when you needed Him— know that He was there, that He still is, and that He has not forsaken you. It is often a trial of our faith to experience what some may call a "disconnect," or feeling silence, from the heavens. These are moments of desperation for many, but if we continue moving forward in faith, we can show our dedication to wanting to know Him.

How can God know the truest intention of our hearts, if He does not test it in all things? He may want to see if we will falter, or stay faithful, when we are unable to hear or feel Him. After these intense trials of faith, floodgates are opened, and more light and knowledge are bestowed upon us. I personally have experienced the trials of silence and disconnect before, and while it was extremely difficult, I remember that the understanding that came afterward was powerful, and moved me to tears of gratitude.

Remember you are eternal. You have always existed, and there has always been trust in *you*. God never falters in His faith in you and your ability to succeed, nor does He doubt your capability to overcome any trial you may face in life. He trusts you *implicitly*— He sent you to earth "trailing clouds of glory."

> *"Our birth is but a sleep and a forgetting:*
> *The Soul that rises with us, our life's Star,*
> *Hath had elsewhere its setting,*
> *And cometh from afar:*
> *Not in entire forgetfulness,*
> *And not in utter nakedness,*
> *But trailing clouds of glory do we come*
> *From God, who is our home:*
> *Heaven lies about us in our infancy!"*

William Wordsworth, Ode:Intimations of Immortality
1770-1850

You are *His* beloved child. He loves you and has not left you to tread these deep waters alone. There are angels around you to bear you up, to lift you and help carry you when you feel you can no longer walk the heavy path to home. Imagine what the world would be like if God never trusted His children! He would never have allowed us to leave His presence. We would not have been granted the opportunity to grow in this lifetime and progress, or obtain Godhood for ourselves. Sheltered and guarded, we would never have been allowed this temporal state to obtain a higher glory. Trust is essential to growth— trust in God is imperative to heal. If we don't completely trust Him, how can we trust in His power to heal us? These are some points to ponder.

When I was completely healed, I was told to cease all supplementation and resume all activities I had done before (including running, which I had been unable to do during my time of illness). I was also encouraged to eat *anything* I wanted in moderation to prove His miraculous power. If I had not trusted in God and His instruction to me, this information could have been really scary! I will admit, there was a split second of concern, but I quickly turned to gratitude and wonder over this miracle, and proceeded forth in faith.

C HAPTER 6

Building the Bridge

In order to heal, there are methodical steps that one must acquire to cross the bridge over the abyss of chronic illness, and reach the safety point of complete healing. This process, when viewed from its entirety, can feel overwhelming and unattainable. When we break it down into small and simple steps, however, it becomes much easier.

"The journey of a thousand miles begins with a single step."
Laozi (604-531 B.C.)

Learning to take the journey ONE step at a time is imperative. One day at a time, knowing you will reach the destination of healing and wholeness, can inspire and lift you as you pursue the path to healing. Everyone's path may look a little different, and no one can know how long it takes. When I became ill, I did not know how long it would take until the resolution, but I knew that resolution would be found. I did not doubt it, and that faith fueled my everyday actions and attitudes. I took it one day at a time, and did not put my own timeline on things. I recognized that it was an opportunity for me to find daily strength and optimism, despite the difficulty of the way. There were darker days and better days, but all the same, I was grateful for the opportunity to be here on earth with my family. I was grateful to have the tools to heal, and the information I needed to proceed. It started with following *one* impression of the Spirit at a time, and then being given another. This way I was not overwhelmed, but continued step by step.

The first step to the healing journey is finding the truth about your illness in the physical sense. If God has placed the truth on the earth about your illness, and it is available to you, you need to seek it out. As we pray in faith to be guided in this matter, we may be prompted to see a certain provider, or study a different modality of healing. We may not immediately receive all the information we need in order to heal, but each encounter we experience is worthwhile. It may not seem so, when you have traversed years of different trajectories and seen so many providers, but it is all for a purpose and reason. I promise you this!

I strongly feel that some of the most benevolent, strongest spirits, took it upon themselves to come down and experience physical and emotional distress. They did so, because others needed an opportunity to learn from them, and expand their own knowledge and understanding. If no one ever was sick, there would be no need of a physician! Health care providers could not learn and grow in the ways they are needed to, without being presented with challenging cases.

I am supremely grateful for every single patient that has come to my office. Because of them, I was able to go and learn, and research and pray, to gain greater insight into the health challenges they were facing. I was able to think outside of the box, knowing that not all the answers were contained in our current medical model. So many of my patients have been patient, as I continued to work, apply new knowledge, and try new modalities, with the deepest desire to help them heal. I would not be the provider I am today without my sweet patients! Truly, it brings such gratitude to my heart, and tears to my eyes, when I think of all their suffering and struggles, and that they were willing to trust me with their care.

To those of you who have suffered for years, and gone to countless providers, and tried countless modalities— I promise you it was not wasted time! During that journey, you have learned patience, persistence, faith, hope, and to not give up. You've developed courage and resolve to do the best you can with what you've received. You've learned to keep trying, to keep getting up, and to keep on going.

Those who have trials of health are some of the most stalwart and stoic individuals, who undergo an incredible refining process to the purification of their souls. It is an honor to know each one of my patients and hear their journeys. I stand in amazement at what they have gone through, and what they have learned through their years of chronic illness. When I learned that the majority of our health problems are created by pathogens, like viruses, bacteria, and toxins, I was thrilled! When I became ill, to find the root cause of the physical manifestation to chronic diseases, was the first step for me in aligning to God's truth in all things.

The second step to the healing journey, is to align to the correct treatment plan once you've identified the root cause to your illness. This includes incorporation of more fruits and vegetables, to let in more light, faith, hope, and love, as well as shifting out foods with fractured spiritual attributes (processed foods with chemicals and additives). This alone makes a marked difference in everyone's constitution and health, even if they don't see immediate results. It can take time to learn how to incorporate this new dietary regime, but you can simplify it by incorporating more whole foods, and making smoothies or simple salads.

When I was bedridden, the easiest things for me to do were to buy frozen fruits, and make a couple smoothies a day, and eat bananas and whole pieces of fruit. I simplified and recognized that food was my medicine, and a foundational piece to helping me heal. The fruit helped my energy levels, mental clarity, and physical strength.

Recognize the adversary will try and dissuade you from eating healthy, making it look too hard or complicated. It does not have to be so! You can reject that unhealthy belief, and make simple changes to incorporate more of these foods into your diet. As you do so, your palate shifts and you begin to crave the deliciousness of fresh produce, and appreciate it for the physical, spiritual, and emotional power it holds to heal you.

I distinctly remember, at one point, eating a lot of papaya daily, as it was very helpful to my symptoms. At first, I begrudgingly consumed it, as I did not like the taste. However, as time passed, I was able to recognize the amazing love it had for me— literally, I could feel its desire to help me on a spiritual level! I became forever grateful for that fruit, and it brings back loving memories now, whenever I eat it.

Fruits and vegetables grow from Mother Earth, in response to the warmth and light of the sun. They grow and produce as God intended, and as such, are full of light and love and gratitude. In their unadulterated state, they are fresh, clean, and delicious to the taste. They literally grow in faith, to weather the storms, winds, and elements. As a result, they can symbolically help us to grow in faith, despite the storms of our lives. When we consume them with gratitude for God's bounty, the power of that fruit or vegetable to nourish us, is increased. The more intention we use in consumption, the greater nutrition (physical, spiritual and emotional) we receive.

If you live in an area with limited access to fresh produce, or your current physical state does not allow a lot of fresh produce due to bowel discomfort, start in small ways. Perhaps canned fruits and vegetables are easier to digest, or dried fruits. As you make the effort to change toward a more nutritious consumption of food, you will be blessed. Praying for those foods to retain a memory of their unprocessed state, also helps boost their nutritional content. Also, if you do not have the funds to purchase organic produce, you can pray in faith, with intention, that negative resonance be removed from your food. Again, Heavenly Father will know what *you* can do to show your faith, and you will also.

Pray to know what you can do to demonstrate your willingness to heal, and act on those spiritual promptings. You may also feel prompted to remove certain foods from your diet, those that do not let in as much light. When we are chronically ill, there are lower energy frequencies, and more darkness in the body. Thus, we have to pull out all the tools of light we possibly can in order to heal and increase in light. Our diet is the foundation to this.

Another part of the correct treatment plan may include specific supplementation. There are innumerable supplements on the market, and many can be helpful. However, often, if we are without clear direction— because we don't know the true cause to our ailment, we will be prone to taking an excess of these that are not necessarily needed. Or we may see some improvement, without a full resolution to our symptoms. This brings about frustration, as so much money is spent on these supports over time, and we can feel like we are getting nowhere.

It is important to know the root cause of your illness, in order to appropriately manage your care plan, and decipher what supplementation will be helpful. God does not want us to go into mountains of debt. He knows what your financial status is. However, it is wise to go over your budget in prayer, and see what you are able to dedicate towards improving your diet, and incorporating specific supplementation if it feels right. Then proceed accordingly. If you truly cannot afford the best quality supplementation, praying over the ones you can afford, so that their potency and absorption is increased, will be acknowledged. Additionally, asking that negative resonance be removed from your supplements or medications, can be a powerful way to eliminate any additives that are not conducive to healing your body.

If funds are limited, focusing on dietary changes and spiritual development, will be the greatest key to your healing journey. You will still reap the benefits of healing when you do all *you* are able to do, in order to demonstrate your faith to heal. This care plan should be developed between you, your provider, and God. Once your care plan is developed, I would encourage you to pray over it, that you will be able to adhere to it, and be guided to make changes when necessary.

You need to receive confirmation that the diagnosis and the care plan are correct for you at this time before you proceed forth. Having that confirmation will help you stick with it through the ups and downs of the healing journey. At times, you may feel that a prescription medication is necessary to provide immediate relief and support, while you are working to tackle the bigger picture. If this occurs, discuss it with your healthcare provider, and pray that they will be directed to the appropriate medication best suited to your needs. This can help prevent multiple failed trials of medications.

There may be additional modalities you feel prompted to incorporate. Some of these include massage, counseling, Christ-centered energy healing, emotional release work, essential oils, acupuncture, acupressure, chiropractic care, and more. All of these are available, and can bring more light into our bodies, when they are directed by the Holy Spirit, and done by a competent, well-trained practitioner. If you feel prompted to explore any of these modalities, be sure to do so in prayer and discernment. Have an open heart and mind, and allow the Spirit to direct you. Having preconceived notions or ideas, or negative beliefs based on another's opinion, will not serve you well. It is imperative that you go in prayer to God, and ask if a certain modality would be beneficial to you, then proceed forth in faith.

I have realized that as God loves all of His children, He has inspired many practitioners to incorporate a variety of healing modalities that can benefit his children. What may work for one individual may not help another. As you have been given dominion over your soul, you will be blessed to know what works for you. Realize that *your* faith is essential for the efficacy of a modality to benefit you.

Once you have recognized the root cause to your physical illness, and incorporated the appropriate treatment plan, the next step is to understand the spiritual cause to your illness. At times, we are given trials of illness to help us grow in faith, hope, and determination. Sometimes illness occurs because of negative emotions, beliefs, experiences, or situations. In simplistic terms, illness sometimes manifests physically because of spiritual or emotional discord. It can be something as simple as unbelief, or avoidance of an important prompting. It can be more complex, such as not forgiving another, or not forgiving yourself in a certain situation.

The more the root of negativity grows, the greater the branches will become. Thus, you begin to incorporate more false beliefs, such as not being good enough, or not being strong enough, or that you are a bad person, etc. These false beliefs will keep being fed to you by the adversary until you are able to recognize the root cause of the spiritual darkness, and remove it from your being, with the help of Christ through repentance.

An example of a root could be a child who was frequently verbally abused, or belittled by an authoritative figure. This situation planted the seed of "I am not good enough," into the heart of the child. As the child grows, the seed grows too, and becomes a tree with branches of regret, remorse, poor self-esteem, lack of confidence, anger, disgust, distrust, envy, and more. The adversary thus latches onto those branches, and feeds the individual with more of the same. They may begin to feel hopeless, and believe nothing will ever change. Yet, the initial cause was a negative belief of not being good enough.

When you can isolate the beginning root cause of all the other emotions, you can hand it over to the Lord in prayer, and let Him take the entire tree away, by getting at the root. Thus, as you work with God to find the root cause to your illness in the spiritual sense, you may be guided and directed to repent of certain things, anything that has separated you from God, that you have incorporated from the adversary. This becomes a liberating exercise, wherein you feel lighter and brighter, and wish to continue seeking out more dark roots, and turning them over to Him.

The more you do this, the more you align to God's will for you, as He wants you to be happy, full of light, and energetic. He knows your potential within, and He wants to help you see that! Yet, if we don't get rid of the roots of darkness, the branches will continue to remain, and overshadow our desires to heal. I cannot underscore this concept enough. There is always a spiritual component to healing the physical frame. One cannot isolate a physical manifestation and think it is separate from the spirit. At times, a medication or other modality can be incorporated, which may bring temporary relief, but if there is a recurring pattern of illness, something deeper needs to be addressed on the spiritual or emotional level.

As we work to address and understand the spiritual aspects to our physical manifestation of illness, we will be guided and directed to do those things that will bring more light into our soul. This again, includes repenting (which also grows our faith), forgiving ourselves and others, serving others, reading God's words, praying, pondering, meditating, listening or singing uplifting music, writing down impressions of the Spirit in a journal, and other exercises as dictated by the Holy Spirit.

To fully heal, we need to incorporate the physical and spiritual aspects of healing, thus addressing the emotional aspect as well. These faith-promoting activities are essential to anyone who has undergone years of chronic illness. Long-term illness has the potential to wear down our fortress of faith and goodwill, and break down our attitude of optimism. We need to daily dedicate the time to filling our vessel with the light of heaven, from whence we came. At the closing scenes of this world, we will not be able to heal without the power of God. He is the only power through which we can conquer every foe, and bring victory to our soul. His son, Jesus Christ, is the ultimate bridge builder! He who saved us from the brink of spiritual and physical death, created a bridge across the chasm of chaos of the soul, to bring us safely home to our Heavenly parents. The way is provided, stretching out before us— but are we willing to take the first step to come home? Are we willing to do our best to show our desires to follow Him, along the path to complete wholeness and healing?

"If thou believest in the redemption of Christ thou canst be healed."
Alma 15:8

If we truly believe in Christ's sacrifice, and that by it, we can be made whole, then we can obtain the promise of being healed in *this* life (if not appointed unto death), through our faithfulness. This can be a literal or spiritual restoration to health. When I researched the historical meaning of health, I was amazed at the diverse explanations for its usage. In old English, the word health meant deliverance, salvation, and healing power. It also meant safety in biblical times. When we consider the role of our Savior in bringing us health— it takes on new meaning upon examination of these definitions.

As we fully accept the Lord's sacrifice in our lives through faith, repentance, baptism, and reception of the Holy Ghost, we are empowered to receive blessings of health and wholeness, and rescued from the powers of the adversary. What a beautiful bridge He has built for us, to cross over to safety and into the loving arms of those who will welcome us on the other side. To never sever ties again with friends and family, and to be complete with them, will be an incredible blessing indeed.

> *"But He was wounded for our transgressions, he was*
> *bruised for our iniquities: the chastisement of our peace*
> *was upon him; and with his stripes we are healed."*
> Isaiah 53:5

When I think of Christ's sacrifice and suffering of my life experiences, it brings me great humility and gratitude, that He would take my pains upon himself, because of His great love for me. As I recognized this sacrifice meant I was worthy to save, it gave me greater understanding into my infinite worth as a child of God. How incredibly important we are in the sight of our Heavenly parents! They love us beyond measure, and they want us to come home to them. The bridge has been built, and the way is prepared to receive complete healing and wholeness. May we build our own bridges to health and healing, through the power of our Savior Jesus Christ, by aligning to the truth behind our illness, and demonstrating our faith to heal.

CHAPTER 7

Light

*"Then spake Jesus again unto them, saying, I am the
light of the world: he that followeth me shall not walk
in darkness, but shall have the light of life."*
John 8:12

What is light? In essence, light is the absence of darkness. In physics, we know there are various degrees of wavelengths of light (or vectors) that create a frequency. Like a radio station, the broader the channel, the easier it is to tune in to. Similarly, a broader wave pattern, or frequency of light, brings more brightness. The brightest light is the light that comes directly from God, and we are told that all truth (light) comes from God. We learn from scriptural accounts, that a man cannot be physically in the direct presence of God, or He would be blown to dust!

*"For behold, I could not look upon God, except his glory
should come upon me, and I were transfigured before him. But
I can look upon thee in the natural man. Is it not so, surely?"*
Moses 1:13

I love this scripture, which is an excerpt of a conversation between Moses and the adversary. After being in the presence of God— and being changed first, so he could behold God's glory and all His creations, Moses then is tempted by Satan. Recognizing the vast difference between the glorious, inconceivable light of God, versus the adversary, Moses has no desire to follow the adversary.

Basically, Moses says to Satan, "Who are you compared to God? Why would I want to follow you?" Such an impressive display of strength, to reject the false beliefs of the adversary, can only come when we obtain a glimpse into the greatness of God's light.

"The glory of God is intelligence- or in other words, light and truth."
Doctrine and Covenants 93:36

How did God obtain His light? He did it little by little, growing in intelligence. Intelligence, is knowledge of truth, and its application in a variety of different planes. Therefore, our Heavenly Father has gained an incredible amount of knowledge and intelligence through experience in a spiritual— then physical, plane as we are doing. Thus, the more *we* experience and learn, the more we grow in light. The more difficult and dark our trials, the more opportunity to grow in intelligence— and light! Also remember, the more light we acquire, the more able we are to cast out the darkness of disease.

It depends on how we manage our trials, as to what amount of light we will obtain as a result. When we understand this concept of light and knowledge, it helps broaden our vision, and empowers us to act accordingly. We can ask God to help us obtain as much light from our trial of health as possible. Doing so, will guide us to build our knowledge from experience, learn new concepts, build upon past experiences, and create things anew. Everything that we create in love and light will bring more of the same back to us, and it glorifies God. We can obtain more intelligence daily, as we pray and seek it out, with help from the Holy Spirit. We can obtain more light, yes, even to the glory of God!

This magnitude of light is inspiring, and incredible to think about. Before any man can see the full power or glory of God, He first needs to be changed. This is the process of turning ourselves to Christ and employing spiritual epigenetics through repentance. Using faith and works to demonstrate our willingness to change, being able to trust in Him completely and wholly, and following the promptings of the Holy Spirit, all affect spiritual gene expression. It allows light to come in from above and blot out any darkness emitting from the "chapters" of our life.

We cannot obtain light on our own, and we can't acquire the purest light without the help of a mediator. Having any bit of darkness within, will diminish the reflection of our light. We cannot stand in front of God without being changed, becoming clean every whit. This alteration comes through the Atonement of Christ, through which all blessings and light flow.

Jesus Christ transcribed everyone's DNA in perfection, which allowed Him to be the coauthor and editor of our chapters, in the ladder of life. He wrote a perfect book (by living a perfect life) so He could edit everyone's "chapters" to perfection. This was done in *every* cell of his body, as our books of life (spiritual DNA) lined up for transcription. He transcribed our pain, worry, sorrow, sins, anger, illness, and every other negative emotion and experience, abridging our chapters to perfection. As he did this, He eliminated all the heartache, pain, sorrow, and illness. He experienced *each* event as we perceived and felt it, to the depths. He also endured the ripple effect of our actions— cascading into those we hurt or injured by our choices. The pain and suffering were so great as he transcribed and translated our experiences that His sweat became great drops of blood. We cannot begin to comprehend the severity of His suffering.

"Which suffering caused myself, even God, the greatest of all, to tremble because of pain, and to bleed at every pore, and to suffer both body and spirit – and would that I might not drink the

*bitter cup and shrink- Nevertheless, glory be to the Father, and I
partook and finished my preparations unto the children of men."*
Doctrine & Covenants 19:18

His work is already done— the books are written in perfection,
but do we allow Him to be a coauthor of our book of life? He is only
able to do this if we allow Him, if we are willing to direct Him to the
chapters wherein healing needs to take place. Historical baggage and
personal dilemmas can be purged from our books, and redirected into
positive emotions, and enduring light. What a glorious realization!
Who does not wish to be healed of every physical, emotional, or
spiritual ailment?

In order to be made whole, we must seek healing on *every* plane,
and wait patiently on the Lord, while we work at this process to
obtain sufficient faith to be healed by His hand. We must seek out
the brightest, truest light of God— His truth in all things.

*"But they that **wait upon the Lord** shall renew their strength;
they shall mount up with wings as eagles; they shall run
and not be weary; and they shall walk and not faint."*
Isaiah 40:31

Acquiring any degree of light is helpful, but for true healing, we
must attain His direct light. We are told that all truth comes from
God, through Christ, the Mediator. Therefore, the more of God's
truth we find, and align to, in *every* topic of study and contemplation,
the more light we will receive. Like a radio station, we want to hone
in on the right frequency— perfect truth, and avoid the static and
dissuading voices of others.

Sometimes the truth of a matter is hard to encounter, because
of the expanse of free thought, and the many hypotheses and ideas
of others. So much information is out there, and so much of it is
incorrect. Like honing in on the right radio station, it may take time
to tune in perfectly and eliminate the static, but when you find it, you

know it. You can *feel* truth in your heart and mind, and it elevates and inspires you. The more truth you know and experience, the easier it becomes to find more, and assimilate it into your life.

Complete truth and light on this earth is meant to be difficult to find, because the path of faithfulness must be *deliberate*. Yet, starting out with as much intelligence of truth that you have, and seeking to add more light to your soul, will guide you to brighter and brighter sources of perfect truth. Like a lighthouse in a distance, seeing it from afar you follow its rays— and are directed to the exact place of its origin. Thus it is with the truth in this world— it will lead you to Christ, and fill you with light— healing both body and soul.

God is deeply vested in our outcome, but justice also resides above. We cannot get "something for nothing"— that is a falsehood to the universe. Just as one electron is given and received between atoms, exchange must occur between God and us. This does not mean we are able to give Him even one billionth back of what He has bestowed upon us, but it does mean we are required to work for more light, and share that light with others in exchange. He knows what we can sacrifice to demonstrate faith. He knows our limitations. We can come to the same deduction of what is required from us by asking in prayer, and following promptings of the Holy Spirit. This is the pattern for growth, as a challenge arises, we seek to know what we are to learn from it, and how we are to act to bring about its resolution.

Man has tried to imitate the light of God. There are advances in harnessing energy of nuclear fission and fusion, that hold promise to be an answer of giving light and warmth to the world. While this pursuit can be noble and good, it discounts the power of God. He is the true source of light. He cannot be replaced by a massive generator, or any other invention that purports to be His equal. Without His light and love, this world would cease to exist.

One of the smallest manifestations of God's light in creation is our sun. This sun is powerful to bring light and warmth to the earth. It is massive and glorious to us, but it is not even a *centesimal* part of His overall light and creation. Because of God, alterations of artificial light have been achieved, but it is never going to be enough to produce long lasting, eternal light. We cannot depend on artificial light to save us in the end— it will not heal our souls. It will be the light of Christ and God, that will lead us home to be healed. We need to discern between His light, and artificial light, to know which path to follow.

Artificial light utilizes similar concepts and laws of natural light, but is seeking to harness and control it. As God has command of the universe, His ability to lovingly direct light and life to the entire world freely, is magnified beyond our understanding. This command of light is done with love, and not by coercion, and is given to us wholly without restraint. Because of the depth of God's perfect love for us, the universe obeys His word, and the sunshine is continuous.

The most brilliant light incorporates all frequencies, amplitudes and wavelengths. The brightest white light is perceived, when all spectrums of color are saturated equally, and projected toward the retina of our eye. This is symbolic of the degree of intelligence and knowledge God has attained. Having descended below all things and ascended above all things (rays of the spectrum), His comprehension of *everything* is expansive. Each topic of study, He has learned and understood to its full depth and breadth, through His own experience. He did not obtain it without personal achievement and serious sacrifice.

This vastness of knowledge had to be acquired over thousands, if not millions of years— yet to Him, time is nothing. The past, present, and future is before Him— all His creations and glory is constantly shining forth. It reflects through Him, making His sight glorious. We saw His glory and brightness before this world was, and it was His light that inspired us to learn and grow as He has done. We desired to become like Him, and we were willing to leave His presence to obtain more light of our own. However, we could not do it alone; and thus, divine help was provided, so we could be guided and directed, using our agency to follow the Holy Spirit.

Christ's sacrifice made it possible for the Holy Spirit to direct His light to each of us. It is what helps us find our path home. For each of us, the quest may start out on a broader road and at a slower pace, but it can progress more quickly toward our Maker. It is dependent upon our faith and trust in Him, as to how and when that will happen. Achieving this light means that we are filling our own vessel with light continually, through *every* source of truth we know. Reading scriptural text, making and keeping covenants with God, and finding His truth in all things (all subjects and studies), lead us toward this light.

The more light we receive, the more we desire it, and the more we are willing to seek out more truth. Yet, the most important truth to find first, is the path home to God— all other truth is circumscribed to it. This path brings with it an abundance of daily spiritual light that will fill our soul, and heal us of our pain and sorrow. We can count on this light to fill us daily, as we strive with all our hearts to obtain His truth.

The light of Christ is a light within every individual, whether they know it or not. It is a light that guides and directs us to truth, and connects us to God. It provides the faith (promoter regions) in our DNA, so transcription can take place in our spiritual DNA everyday. Without His light, we would be unable to act, to choose and proceed, in one way or the other. Like a spiritual tether, it provides us with added support and direction, when we feel stuck or lost. It helps to prompt us to action, and to pursue something we had never before considered or explored. It brings with it a clarity that sustains us during the most perilous and difficult times, and provides peace amidst the struggle. This light is a frequency that cannot be forged, or proven to existence, by man's knowledge. It is a knowledge that must be gained by the Spirit. Like a burning fire within our heart, it ignites the individual's spirit and gives them more power and courage to continue on, despite the length of their healing journey.

The light of Christ is like the sun. It sustains, warms, and provides life to this planet. It grants us with the ability to see everything around us for what it is, and helps us avoid dangerous terrain and hazardous situations. It brings seeds to germination, so that they may spring forth as plants, flowers, and shrubs. The plants then provide animals with sustenance, as well as us.

I find it so fascinating that the sun is *always* shining! Indeed when we are in the darkness of the night, it is merely because we are abiding in the shadow of the earth. (Dieter F. Uchtdorf, "Bearers of Heavenly Light," *Ensign* or *Liahona*, Nov. 2017) Therefore, darkness is merely the absence of God's light. At night, the sun's rays still reflect off the moon, giving us the lesser light. It is a reminder that the sun is still present and always giving light and warmth. We, on earth, are the ones who turn away from the sun into the shadow of darkness. Thus, symbolically, we can remove ourselves from the spiritual shadows, and stand joyfully in the sun's rays. They will cleanse, purify, and heal us, as we bask in the sun's warmth and love.

The sun also has medicinal properties for us! It prevents the growth of harmful bacteria and viruses. It also destroys pathogens on the skin, in the blood, and in mucous membranes. Currently, research has focused on UV radiation to kill pathogens, but the reality is, the energy of the sun's rays is sufficient to kill them! When we do not have access to medications, supplements, or other therapies to heal, the sun can be the most beneficial weapon to combat illness!

When I was healed, one of the most powerful meditations leading up to this was regarding the sun. I would literally imagine myself going straight up into space, and standing directly in front of the sun! I would imagine the sunlight permeating my being, from the crown of my head, all the way down to my toes. I would absorb as much light as I was able to, and when a new symptom came up somewhere else in my body, I would send sunlight there. I found as I did this, my discomfort went away, and the darkness of disease disappeared. My pain resolved, and my strength improved. This can be your reality too!

The sun also can heal us, by providing the means, whereby, our body can synthesize vitamins and minerals essential to health, that are unknown to current science and research today. On your journey to ultimately heal, regard the power of the sun. Meditate about the sun, and include sunlight in your life. This light, and its warmth, will sustain you during your darkest trials of health.

Another perspective of light, is the "absence of heaviness." When we are going through an incredibly difficult trial of our health, we often feel heavy and weighed down. We feel like we can't go on another day in this misery, and we may feel hopeless or depressed. We may desire to give up completely, and not continue on— but we cannot give in to this ideology! The negative emotions would like to enter in and drag us down, to keep us in sickness and misery. But we can choose to turn to light, and make the best of our situation, by keeping things "lighter."

Laughter is truly the best medicine, and finding ways to incorporate laughter into our lives, despite the difficulty of the way, is incredibly helpful. At one point, I came up with images of me suffering in my head, and then imagined something comical occuring, like falling down the stairs— as if it couldn't get any worse right?! I had to make light of the difficult situations encountered in my life.

For another example, I would imagine a woman in a coma in the ICU. As a nurse, I would enter the room and look around, calling for Prince Charming to show up, so we could wake her immediately. Another visual "joke" was viewing someone who was bleeding profusely. I would attend to them and ask, "Are you type A? Because if you are, you've got a handle on this already." Rather than referencing their blood type, I was in reality referencing a type A personality— which I myself have been! It is truly helpful to come up with comical images or jokes that will make you laugh!

There were times I was in such misery that my soul just began to laugh! I laughed so hard on many occasions, that I started to cry in laughter, because the pain and sorrow were so profound. Laughter raises our energy frequency to a level at which we can heal. As we discuss frequency— vibrational waves of light, it brings about more understanding of how positive emotions such as laughter, will fill us with more light, and diminish the darkness. Helping others to laugh, as well, is comfort to our soul, and brings healing to you and others, and the effect of healing is magnified. If you have a jokester in your midst, you are blessed! Welcoming a wholesome prank that brings laughter is a blessing.

We also think of light as illumination— understanding and knowledge gained. This perspective of light ties back to the importance of finding the truth of God in all things. The more knowledge and understanding we can gain of Him, and His plan for each of us individually and collectively, the greater light we can receive from above. As we search out His light from various sources, we will be able to hone in more and more on the purest, brightest light of His love, and be completely healed.

As you think of a spectrum of light, with varying degrees into darkness— aim for the brightest light you can think of. Follow its guiding path, and it will bring you home to healing. At times, we may be required to learn and grow through experience, sorting through the information available to us. We then are encouraged to retain the true portion, and discard the remainder. Asking for God to "shed light" on the topic of study, so that the true portion will stand out to you, is essential during these times.

"To light" something, is a verb indicating igniting something, as a fire. Truly, in the furnace of affliction, we become a refined individual, stronger and more resilient to the trials around us. We learn to rely on power from above, and strengthen our foundation of faith.

> *"If the foundation of faith is not embedded in our*
> *hearts, the power to endure will crumble."*
> (Henry B. Eyring, "Mountains to Climb,"
> *Ensign* or *Liahona*, May 2012)

It is important that we do not let our light go out! A burning flame can be extinguished by raindrops of doubt, fear, disbelief, distrust, frustration, impatience, or selfishness. If we have been fortunate enough to develop a flame of faith, we can continue to feed it with optimism, hope, trust, belief, patience, and service. It has to *continually* be given the kindling of positivity, on which to thrive and grow. Thus, the flame becomes a growing fire that cannot be extinguished, emitting greater light and warmth.

We can bring warmth, sustenance and hope to others when we become lit with the flame of faith, and continue to employ the virtues from which it grows. This process is only made available through the power of Jesus Christ. Because He blotted out the negative from our books of life, we can beseech Him to be our coauthor and produce our greatest work. Our book of life can be a beacon of light to all who will be invited to read it one day.

CHAPTER 8
Charity and Divine Love

*"Greater love hath no man than this, that a
man lay down his life for his friends."*
John 15:13

I find it fascinating that God loved all His children so much, He was willing to let us leave His presence, and come to this earth. He recognized the importance of agency for our growth, and thus allowed us to leave our Heavenly home. Yet, He did not leave us without guidance. By His love, we were granted the light of Christ, the influence of the Holy Spirit, help of angelic hosts, and a plethora of other tools to help us remember our purpose here. Indeed, He desired that we all could return to His presence, and so He provided the way. He thus demonstrated the greatest act of love in sending His only begotten Son as a sacrifice for the world.

Because of our love and faith in Christ pre-mortally, and *His* reciprocal love for us, He was able to complete the most difficult, arduous, and tormenting journey from Gethsemane to Golgotha. Because of His love for us, we can be clean every whit, made whole, and healed, through the power of the Atonement. Our spiritual DNA can be shifted and altered to its perfect state, and become full of His light. This kind of love, and its reciprocation, goes beyond mortal understanding. Have you ever considered what would have happened had Christ not completed His mission? We would have been eternally lost to ruin and decay, never receiving resurrection or eternal progression! All our experience here would be for naught without a Redeemer. The magnitude of this redemptive power from any spiritual, physical, and emotional blow, could only be founded on the principle of divine love.

Divine love provides the strongest, most unbreakable bond in eternity, by which the Atonement was created. Christ's perfect love in our Father instilled in Him humility, patience, kindness, forgiveness, service, and a willingness to submit to all things in His life— including false judgment, ridicule, and physical and emotional affliction. His perfect love for us allowed Him to endure well the depths of pain and hell, and be restored to a fullness of joy and glory. Indeed, it has helped me endure the trials of this life, when I ponder His eternal example. The depiction of this love is revolutionary, but how do we obtain it?

In order to understand this love, we must first know our Heavenly Father. As we seek to know our Heavenly Father in earnest, He fills us with a measure of His love. We are thus able to love Him in return, and comprehend more the depth of divine love. Indeed, we cannot feel the full amount of His love for us in our physical state, because it would be too overpowering. But we can rest assured that His love is equal in power and potency to Christ's.

> *"For the Father loveth the Son, and sheweth him*
> *all things that himself doeth: and he will shew him*
> *greater works than these, that ye may marvel."*
> John 5:20

As Christ came, and did everything He had seen the Father do, we can know that He loves us *as* deeply as our Heavenly Father. We can look to His example to further understand God's love for us.

I have a dear friend who shared her experience with me of feeling God's love. She reports that she had been in the woods to pray, and connect with God. Initially, she did not feel anything positive, and she was discouraged. But later that day, she had a remarkable experience where she was filled to capacity with God's love for her. His love was so consuming, so powerful, that she could not move, and it filled her with such joy, such gratitude and peace, that she could not stop crying. She remembers understanding it was only a spec of God's love for her— because if she was allowed to feel it all, she would have exploded. My friend was forever changed from that one small moment, by experiencing a fraction of God's love for her.

Here in the mortal realm, we are not initially equipped to handle such a magnitude of emotion. Our capacity to understand and demonstrate love, may be diminished by the veil that blocks recollection of our previous existence. Yet, it is part of our journey here to uncover that deep and abiding love of God, self, and others, that we can only receive through Christ. It is the most rewarding, and difficult, concept to learn here on earth— to love as Christ loves. Love in action is Charity- the pure love of Christ.

How can we develop charity toward ourselves? Indeed, the world is full of ideologies that inhibit our ability to love ourselves, as children of God. We are taught by the world, that we can't love ourselves and be content, unless we look and act a certain way, or have certain material things. Some individuals, particularly women, often feel that they need to give, and give, and give— without taking care of themselves, to gain acceptance. This causes them to become burnt out, and depleted. It is a martyr-like approach that has become a socialized expectation.

Somehow, women and men often feel the need to meet societal expectations that may be wholly incongruent with God's design. If such worldly ideals are not met, self worth plummets to the ground. On the contrary, some individuals love themselves over God, and this too, is a deception. "Selfie sticks" have been heralded in to demonstrate this point (pun intended). Individuals become enamored with achievement, stature, and financial gain, and forgo asking what *God* wants them to do. Instead, they seek to obtain only what *they* want. They place themselves on the pedestal of worldly success, while kicking the founder of their fortune to the curb— and become a servant of the adversary. Where is the balance?

How can we love ourselves, without becoming selfishly involved? As we seek our Father and His will for us, we are granted knowledge of our divine worth and purpose. We feel and understand the redemptive power of Christ that can bring us back to their presence. We understand our role with them, and how we can overcome all things through Christ. This brings appreciation of ourselves, as a creation of God, and grows gratitude within for all we have. That gratitude then springs into respect, reverence, and love for who we are, and what we can become. When this transpires, we see *others* for their potential, and can love them more perfectly. We become a bearer of heavenly light, and are able to transmit His love and light to others. Thus charity begins to bloom.

"He that hath my commandments and keepeth them, he it is
that loveth me: and he that loveth me shall be loved of my Father,
*and I will love him, and will **manifest myself to him**."*
John 14:21

How can we truly exemplify charity? How can we obtain it? We first must give Christ our love, which is then reflected back to us, and purified through Him. How do we give our love to Him? *By keeping his commandments.* Literally, divine power is unlocked within us, as we obey the laws that bring us into alignment with Him. We are blessed to know Him with even more familiarity, as we go through trial and tribulation, praying for His guidance and obeying His will.

We also understand more the depth of Christ's love, when we have been forgiven of past wrongs, delivered from our addictions or temptations, or guided to an answer we were seeking. We become more aware of Him in our lives, as we observe the *daily* tender mercies, that let us know He is real. It could be the helpful cashier at checkout, or a friend just stopping by to say hello.

Even a brilliant sunrise, or gorgeous sunset, is a demonstration of His love for us. Things that are orchestrated so perfectly in their timing, remind us that God is aware of us, and it is a supernal way He shows us His love. As we seek for the little daily miracles and tender mercies, we grow in gratitude to God. This allows us to receive more light and love into our spiritual DNA. Gratitude is the catalyst of love, and it causes us to act. There are many genes of gratitude, and the more we have— the better off we will be.

An incredible tender mercy is to have a family on this earth. To receive a family is another manifestation of God's love for us. It also brings with it, an invitation to comprehend more of God's love. As a brother, sister, spouse, parent, or child, each of us has the opportunity to cultivate love in our family, and make sacrifices for the welfare of others. Parents are expected by God to love their children, and teach them truth. Spouses are expected to love and honor one another, with complete fidelity and trust. As we seek to do these things as a family, we strengthen each other, and support personal potential and growth.

Every family is different, and may be differently comprised, due to circumstance and situation, but all of us can strive to grow together in a loving environment. Each of us, has a responsibility to create peace and harmony, and a safe space for healing. If your circumstance has not been as favorable growing up, due to the agency of others, you are not alone, and you are not forgotten. Angels witness your life from birth to death. Anything that is not rightfully given, will be granted to you in due time— either later in this mortality, or after this life, through the Atonement of Christ.

As we are all children of God, indeed, on a grander scale, we all are family! We can choose to view each other as divine offspring with the same parentage, and likewise, seek to lift and love others. There may be difficulties and disunion at times in our family setting, but love allows us to seek resolution of such conflicts. This love promotes patience, forgiveness, fairness, mercy, selflessness, and compassion, as we go through life together.

Without this principle of divine love, families can fall to the wayside, and divisiveness may manifest. When we forgo filling ourselves with God's love and light, we lose our power to manifest it to others. It is thus imperative, that we seek our Savior *daily*, to avoid the darkness of deception and decay. As we reflect on His words and the acts of His life, we will retain a remembrance of His divine love, and transcribe it in our spiritual DNA. This will change our gene expression, and we will become more loving towards ourselves, and others.

This is why Christ came to this earth, and His teachings were recorded. Our Father wanted His example of love for us to follow, and learn from. One cannot include all the contents of scripture that relate to Christ's perfect love in just one book— indeed, volumes of books could not contain all writings regarding this topic! His presence, ministering, miracles, and words were all a manifestation of divine love. His ability to coauthor our book of life, through our own repentance, is only possible through Christ's atoning sacrifice. His is a sacrifice that transcends time; it is available to all who have lived or will yet live on this earth. It surpasses space, and all realms of existence. It is incomprehensible to man, but perfectly positioned by God.

As we are all divine beings, humanity as a whole has demonstrated love throughout history. We are inspired by stories of individuals who went out of their way to serve, or who made great sacrifices to rescue others. Many have sacrificed their lives for love of their country and fellow man, and even more so, for God. Because of love, we have homeless shelters, food banks, refugee assistance programs; campaigns to raise money for school supplies, shoes and other necessities, and to provide clean running water in underserved areas.

We open doors for others, smile and say hello, and offer donations when tragedy or natural disaster strike. As a whole, the human race possesses a great capacity to love one another. This capacity will be magnified as we seek to align to Christ, by following His ways. When we do this, our spiritual DNA, as a whole, will shift much more rapidly toward the blueprint of our Heavenly parents.

Despite the innate goodness of humankind, there is an adversarial force that some have chosen to follow. The enticements of control, lust, and greed have replaced the swelling emotions of divine love and virtue in their hearts. They hide from shame, initially, until they become numb to it, and continue down a damned path. These individuals seek power, and have damaged lives, and broken trust, among those who loved them. They are insatiable in their appetite for false love and adoration, and use a variety of means to trick and manipulate others, leaving a wake of disappointment and disillusionment behind them.

These poor individuals have chosen to cut themselves off from the love of God— and their DNA is deadening. This corrupted idea of love comes from a desire to manipulate and control others, instead of granting them agency and mercy— and is all selfishly based. Often, this type of false love or allegiance is maintained by bribery, threats, fear, physical injury, emotional torment, and blatant disregard for another's well-being.

Those who have been injured by this *false* idea of love, may have received a skewed experience, and therefore, find difficulty embracing and understanding how to receive love. Their past experiences can literally encode the DNA in reverse fashion, and inhibit their ability to accept and recognize Christ's love— or the love of anyone else. This is often why individuals return to the same abusive relationship, or continue in dysfunctional ones.

Our perception of love is programmed into the very cells of the body. If you have been burdened by experiences of false love, abuse, or neglect, recognize that this is *not* the true source of real love. Man's attempt to control love is a mockery to God, and brings down those who would choose to use it as thus. You *cannot* control divine love, as it has no bounds.

There are no requirements for this type of love, no amount of service or stature you must reach to receive this love. It has no price, it is granted to *you* merely because you are part of creation, *and* you seek to follow God's laws. This type of love is infinite, and holds no bounds; it is all encompassing, and can enclose and remove *any* imperfection or vice if we let it. This love is where we came out of creation, to grow and develop into eternal newness.

If you have frustration, heartache, and hurt from past experiences, but long to receive the love of God— come to your Savior! He has the power to heal all wounds, to dispel the doubt and regret, to silence painful memories and filter negative emotions, and to remove triggers from recurring events. His love is so magnificent, even one tiny spec of this love would fill your soul to bursting. Often, when emotionally injured by another, we block our hearts to prevent any negative emotion from harming us further. However, in so doing, we often become numb to the very emotions that would heal our heart completely! It may seem scary at first, but removing the blockade around our heart, is essential to allowing the love of God into our souls. We can do this through sincere prayer, and by asking for our heart to be open to His love.

When we allow the love of our Heavenly Father into our souls, we *heal* deep spiritual and emotional wounds, which then transmits to physical healing. We begin to receive confidence to stand our ground, and disallow anyone to injure us again, because we genuinely know our true worth from God. We live with our heart, and are not concerned with what others may think or say. As we do this, we gain a greater measure of this love and light, and can transmit it to others.

To receive this love, we *must* turn our heart over to God, and allow Him to heal it, and make it whole through Christ. We must be willing to do what *He* wants us to do, and not seek out our own agenda. We need to be willing to give His love freely to others, and without restraint. We can become a conduit through which His love can flow to others, and, in turn, it purifies our souls. The more we give this love to others, the greater amount we receive in return, from heaven.

As God's love is infinite, there will always be more available than we can ever give. Yet, it allows us opportunities for growth and understanding, that could come in no other way. When we strive to mirror Jesus Christ, We begin to see ourselves as He does. Our countenance begins to be reflected in Him. We begin to understand more our purpose and mission here on earth. We also begin to understand others, when we approach them with love. We see them more clearly for who they are, and know of their potential and goodness.

When we act out of love, we are more likely to be patient, kind, helpful, forgiving, and service oriented. God's love is ever growing and expanding, and being a conduit of His love brings the greatest joy and happiness. When we live from this place of divine love, we are in the highest frequency of healing! The better we can obtain and maintain it, the faster we will heal.

We all want to be on the same progressive path to return home to the safety and love of God. We each have imperfections and weaknesses, but we can recognize that Christ's love makes it possible for us to love one another.

> *"But I say unto you, Love your enemies, bless them that curse you, do good to them that hate you, pray for them which despitefully use you and persecute you"*
> Matthew 5:44

Loving our enemies has been a commandment from the beginning. Yet it is probably the hardest one to obey. It is easy to love someone who reciprocates our love, or even receives it without recoil. Yet to love our enemy, it takes a great act of will to ask that our hearts be changed toward them. The law of justice promotes a mindset of "an eye for an eye," but mercy has a greater claim on our ability to love others— even those who are the most difficult to love.

Loving our enemies does not mean we must voluntarily expose ourselves time and time again to their injurious methods. But it does mean we should pray for them, provide for their needs when they are in want (if we are able), and use kind words in their presence. We need not engage in prolonged conversations of conflict, but allow them their agency and action, without damaging our own dignity. Christ himself, forgave the very men who beat him and nailed him to a cross, yet he did not respond to their taunts and jeering. We too, can likewise be peaceable and kind, to even our very enemies.

Who is our enemy? I believe an enemy can be any*thing* or any*one* that we view with contempt— anything that opposes us, and from whom (or what), we seek refuge. We often think of a person who has wronged us, or injured us, to be an enemy; but have we considered our vices, our weaknesses, or even our physical trials, to be an "enemy"? If we are viewing them in anger, frustration, or contempt, it may be something to consider.

I recall when I was struggling so much with my personal trial of health, there were times I was angry and frustrated. If I allowed myself to think about all the symptoms I was dealing with, and all the difficulty it caused me, I would easily be pulled down into more anger and frustration and darkness. But, if I allowed the viruses to just "do their thing," and didn't focus on them, but instead on serving others, my symptoms weren't as severe, and I was uplifted and more positive. I can now honestly say that I have deep gratitude and love for the pathogens that caused my illness, because they gave me the greatest opportunity to learn, in a way no other thing could.

I recognize now, that I was able to develop patience, persistence, diligence, trust, empathy, forgiveness, charity, more faith, and a whole host of other attributes, by doing my best to stay positive during my prolonged trial of chronic illness. One day, I was encouraged by a friend to write down *all* the blessings I had received through my trial of health. Indeed, I came up with a list of people I'd met, things I'd learned, and what I have understood now physically, emotionally, and spiritually. The list will continue to grow; I am certain, as I reflect back and ponder on the many things I experienced and felt.

If you haven't done so, I would encourage you, at some point, to sit down and reflect, and write down all the blessings you have seen in your life, as a result of your health trial. The list may start out small at first, but it will continue to grow as you keep returning back to it. Viewing this list on a regular basis, will help you through the most difficult times, and in turn, will help others as well.

Is it possible to love pain? Pain is an incredibly difficult adversary to face. No one wants to be in pain, indeed, we all strive to steer clear of it. We may postpone surgeries, or avoid extreme physical exertion, or run away from a blood draw— because we dislike pain. There are many different types of pain. Physical, emotional, and spiritual pain can all drive us to be bitter and angry, if we allow it. However, these discomforts can also encourage us to seek resolution to deeper seeded issues, by praying for guidance from above, while we work on fixing the root causes.

Pain is always an indicator that something needs to be addressed. We can welcome it as a guide to higher healing, or suppress it until it becomes a larger burden to bear. Indeed, we can love pain as an opportunity to grow and learn, and address something of import. Too often, we suppress pain, or mask it with something that does not fix the root cause. This may provide immediate relief, but will not bode well for us long term. This excludes acute physical pain and injury, and surgical intervention, that promotes a need for acute pain relief. Indeed, we are blessed with medications to relieve pain when needed. But we should not solely rely on them if there are other modalities and lifestyle changes we can make to address it more fully.

What is spiritual pain? This is a pain rarely discussed, but is ever so real. It is a feeling of being separated from our Heavenly Parents; a feeling of isolation and loneliness that can be pervasive, despite being surrounded by productivity, and loving friends or family. This separation may feel like home-sickness, despite being "home" on this earth. It may also feel like being lost and directionless, as if your life holds no meaning. It can feel like darkness and emptiness, if we cut ourselves off from God's influence through our choices, and is a manifestation of our conscience.

This is not to be confused with depression, as depression has physical and emotional components to its etiology. This is, indeed, from spiritual separation from our heavenly home. This type of pain can be healed, and complete resolution can be had! It comes as we become aware that we are not separated from them spiritually, and that there is always the opportunity to speak with them. We can seek out their direction to bring us to the path that will lead us back to our heavenly home. We can ask for more faith in them, and to feel their love for us. We can look for the tender mercies— the symbols of their love for us, in our daily life. They are always present and willing to listen, but often, we are the ones who don't come to converse.

Emotional pain may be the hardest to heal from, because the modalities to heal it are not easily understood. This pain derives from traumatic experiences, heartbreak, grief and loss, betrayal, and consequential chaos from our actions or the actions of others. This pain cannot be buried long-term for it will resurface. It must be recognized and addressed for complete healing to occur.

Many individuals turn to cognitive behavioral therapy, which can prove helpful. However, there are other modalities that many are not aware of. Emotional clearing modalities can be hugely beneficial for many individuals. I would encourage you to be open to other modalities, if counseling alone has not proven helpful. Again, the belief you have in a modality can also increase the efficacy, but if you are at a standstill in your progress— it may be an indicator to look outside the box.

I have seen many individuals heal from extreme emotional trauma. Most of them did not do counseling alone, but focused on using other modalities to process and clear emotions, through the atonement of Jesus Christ. They employed meditation and other modalities to hand their emotional burdens over to the Lord and let it go, never to take it back. It can be a process and it takes time, but it can be done.

Filling your life with positivity, and emotions of gratitude, love, and faith, helps to prevent retention of historical hurt and heartache.

I know many of you have gone through hell and back, with certain life experiences. My heart goes out to you, and I ache for you. But I would encourage you not to give up! You are more powerful than you know; you are indeed worth *worlds*! You can overcome and find joy in this life. Finding someone who has successfully cleared emotions from similar circumstances can be extremely helpful.

God will place individuals in your path who are specific to serve you. Be open and aware, as you prayerfully seek out all the options available to heal from emotional turmoil. It often takes a few modalities to help in severe circumstances. And I cannot underscore the emotional support that we receive through fruits and vegetables. Indeed, there are spiritual and emotional attributes to whole foods.

The foods produced from Mother Earth are designed to support us on our sojourn here. They have spiritual, emotional, and physical attributes, and are a foundation to healing from anything! When we shift our diet towards healthier eating, that alone unlocks emotional detox, and can be refreshing and eye opening. We additionally gain greater insight into ourselves, and what we can do to further heal.

I am grateful for pain, as it has become one of my greatest teachers. It alerted me that my body needed help and support. It allowed me to recognize the things I had historically done, that were not beneficial to my health and wellness as a whole. It has helped me realize we are not just a physical persona, but are connected spiritually to a higher power that can help us heal. It allowed me to incorporate other healing modalities I was never aware of before, and opened my eyes to things unseen. It has helped me understand that emotional and spiritual pain, can contribute to physical pain, and vice versa. Moreover, it has taught me that we are stronger than we know, and can overcome *all* things through faith in Jesus Christ, who suffered every caliber of pain. We can, in time, find a friend in pain.

It is important to note that divine love is not unconditional. God always will love us with a perfect love, but that does not mean He can excuse us from anything we say or do. The Universe, and its laws, do not allow this. Indeed, God himself, has dictated the truth of this when Christ said:

"As the Father hath loved me, so have I loved you: continue ye in my love. If ye keep my commandments, ye shall abide in my love; even as I have kept my Father's commandments, and abide in His love."
John 15: 9-10

To "abide in His love" and be with Him eternally, we must obey His commandments, and align to His word. Doing so, empowers us to receive more guidance and direction, and increases our capacity to receive His love. The more love and light we receive from Him—the greater capacity we have to receive healing. As we love others, as He has loved us, and keep His commandments, we are showing our Heavenly Parents that we truly want to become like our Savior, Jesus Christ. And in so doing, we can be healed.

CHAPTER 9

Unity

It is important for us to consider the deep truth that we are part of the Universe. Amid all its intricacies and beauty and endless habitation, we reside. We are eternal, we have always existed, and we will exist still upon cessation of this mortal life. There can be no substitute for a temporal existence, wherein, we learn the truth about our relationship to God.

Indeed, without a physical separation from our Heavenly Parents, we could not develop a deeper connection to them. We couldn't appreciate everything they have done for us, without coming down to partake of the physical temptations and trials they too once experienced. When we recognize that they went through the same process as we, to become who *they* are, it gives us greater faith, hope, and trust, that we too can overcome any trial we face in this life.

> *"God himself was once as we are now, and is an exalted man, and sits enthroned in yonder heavens! ... It is the first principle of the Gospel to know for a certainty the Character of God, and to know that we may converse with him as one man converses with another, and that he was once a man like us; yea, that God himself, the Father of us all, dwelt on an earth, the same as Jesus Christ himself did."*

(*Teachings of the Prophet Joseph Smith,* sel. Joseph Fielding Smith
[1938], 345–46)

Because they once struggled and suffered through their own
mortal experiences, they also know how to succor us. This can bring
us much comfort when we feel we have reached the bottom of our
barrel. I remember first learning about the word succor, and being
overcome with gratitude. To succor means to *run* to someone's aide.
Not to slowly meander or wander, but to directly address their *need,*
immediately.

It is important to remember that God will not always take away
our sorrow, pain, or suffering immediately, because it may *not* be
what we need. But He may strengthen us, and give us more patience
or power to endure by faith, when we feel we can go on no longer. We
came down here to experience physical mortality, so we can become
like our Heavenly Parents! This requires a lot of work and effort. We
can't expect it to be easy. But we *can* trust that God knows what we
need to grow and learn, as He was a mortal himself.

We can understand God's will for us more fully, when we engage
in powerful prayer. Powerful prayer means asking in faith, *only* for
those things the Holy Spirit prompts us to. It is putting off the
natural man— our wants and desires, and instead placing our divine
spiritual self as the mouthpiece to our supplication. This incredible
experience of prayer often ensues when we turn our will over to
the Father, trust His timetable, and open our hearts to receive His
guidance.

We wait patiently for the Holy Spirit to inspire us to request
those things which we *need,* to give us strength and succor during
our health trial. I remember distinctly during my trial of Lyme, that
I did not ask God to heal me, because I hadn't felt prompted to, until
the end of the trial was near. I remember asking everyday for spiritual
gifts that I felt prompted to request, and I expressed gratitude daily—
multiple times a day, for my body, and for the tools I had been given
to help my body heal (healthy foods, supplements, etc). I knew that

there were still things I needed to learn, and through revelation from the Spirit, I recognized the time of complete healing was not yet.

The unity I felt with my Father when I prayed to Him in this manner was astounding. The comfort and love that only a Father can give, enveloped me, and strengthened me. I could literally feel Him wiping away my tears, as I poured out my heart to Him everyday, submitting to His timeline, and doing my best everyday. I remember once learning that, as God has created all things, everything with which we are blessed, comes directly from Him. Thus, we truly can give nothing back to Him— except our agency.

Our will is the *only* thing we can ever give back to our Heavenly Father. That is the only thing He wishes of us. He knows if we submit to His will, we will become like Him. He is all-powerful because He Himself abides by all the laws of heaven with *strict* obedience— and that is what He is trying to teach to us. Obedience to Him and making our will His— brings a unification of our spirits, wherein, we can access God's power to heal. This transcendent blessing is made possible by the atoning sacrifice of our Savior. The vehicle of its transmission comes through the Holy Spirit.

The Holy Spirit promotes unity as it testifies of God's truth. We can learn about why we are here, and where we came from, and what we can achieve in the next life, through scripture. We read about Jesus Christ and His life, His miracles of healing, and His sacrifice and resurrection— all of which were done for our benefit. Yet, we could not fully understand and *feel* the veracity of these things without the Holy Spirit. The Holy Spirit touches our hearts, and teaches us these things are true. It helps direct us to the correct path that leads to eternal life, and even exaltation, as we seek it in earnest.

The Spirit unifies our hearts, as we become one in purpose to do God's will here on the earth, to serve each other, and follow Christ's example. When we recognize this, that we are intimately connected through our suffering, to Christ, miracles happen. We no longer isolate a person in peril, and leave them on the wayside, but we see them for the infinite potential they hold, and we recognize their divinity within. We *know* the power of the Atonement, because we've seen it work in our lives, and know it can do the same for others.

When we can see someone as our brother or sister, with the eye of unwavering faith, we know of a surety they can overcome their weakness through Christ, as can we. Thus, a channel of power is unlocked, and flows down from the heavens to strengthen the individual, and those in service to them. Through our faith in another, they truly can change. Unbreakable faith is infectious, and because we bestow our faith in them, they begin to have faith in themselves.

When others see our incredible faith in them, and feel God's love for them through us, they will eventually want to learn of God. They then learn to love God, and know that through *His* power, any weakness or addiction can be overcome. Because of *His* faith in them, their hearts begin to soften and change, and they no longer desire to live in chaos. They humbly seek out help from God, and He, in turn, sends us as His angels to lift them. Thus begins a unified effort to help each other, which in turn, strengthens and edifies everyone involved. We become unified in gratitude and service by this connection.

When dealing with chronic illness, we are blessed with humility, and are turned to the things that really matter. We forgo worldly cares, and focus on the small and simple things that bring true joy into our lives. We recognize that the most important thing in this life is our relationship with God, family, friends, neighbors, pets, and others. We don't care about the latest trends or fashions, or owning a flashy car— because we recognize that these things hold no lasting joy.

We become supremely grateful for the simplicity of shelter, food, and comfortable clothing, the basic necessities of life. We delight in the sunrise, or the smell of freshly cut grass. Our senses become enlightened, and we notice the beauty of nature around us. We become unified in our relationships, as loved ones seek to lift us in our struggles, and we do likewise for them. This circle of support brings long-lasting joy and gratitude.

We also learn of our relationship to ourselves— how we are

children of God, and He has endowed us with the ability to conquer any misfortunes, or difficulties, we may encounter. When we can realize this truth, and recognize the incredible capacity we possess, our life will change. Becoming one with God allows us to access His power. We literally can feel the energy and frequency of those around us, and therefore, help others progress and turn towards God. Therein is found the beauty of oneness and unity.

There are many different faculties in which oneness can be expressed. When we, as a spirit, are united to our physical body, we learn to become one in that union. Our spirit and our body combined allow us to experience a variety of emotions and circumstances that would otherwise be impossible to acquire. We are able to feel every sensation and hazard of mortality. Our bodies are a working system of organs, receptors, and communication, and each system cannot exist without the other.

We have a heart to pump blood through the vascular system, which then diffuses oxygen and nutrients to tissues. We cannot diffuse oxygen into tissues without the ability to acquire oxygen through the lungs. We cannot send nutrients to the tissue, without absorption of food compounds through the bowel, and we cannot eliminate waste products from the blood, without the function of the kidneys, liver, and lungs.

Through the blood, we transport hormones that act as messengers from organ systems, to communicate and send feedback to the other; thus maintaining homeostasis among all systems in their perfection. Additionally, through the blood we perfuse every tissue— muscle, bone, and sinews, that we may function properly. Without muscle and bone, there would be no structure in which to hold our frame together, and we would fall apart!

We are held together by our sinews. Our experiences and emotions are written on our very sinews. Regard this statement for a moment— if the essence of our being is written on our sinews, and sinews promote unity, what does that signify for us? Sinews are the tendons and ligaments of the body that promote movement and forward progression. They also connect the bones and ligaments in the most perfect way, to allow for mobility and strength in the most efficient matter. Nothing is wasted wherein the sinews are attached and articulated.

The sinews are what promote the unity of the body, and its capacity to excel— and it is representative of our spirituality as well. Collectively, as a body, we are connected by what we think, say or do— it ripples out into the world and affects others in our sphere of influence. We can ask ourselves what are we doing to contribute to unity, and forward progression as a whole? Are our actions and words hindering, or promoting, improvement and progression towards greater unity?

The blood is another connecting factor that delineates this concept of unity. Without the blood, there would be no communication between systems, no waste products removed, no nutrients given, no oxygen distribution. Without the blood, we would be completely and utterly wasted.

This life-blood can be a representation of Heavenly Mother. Her feminine energy is nourishing, detoxifying, and rejuvenating. Reception of her love is essential for our health. Her love comes to us physically, and even spiritually, through Mother Earth— from the plants that grow in her fertile soil. Thus, consumption of whole fruits and vegetables direct from their source, cleans our blood, and allows Her love to travel freely within us. The more we can receive her love, in gratitude for the food that she provides, the greater our health will be.

As the body is created with so much love and care, it demonstrates every form of unity known to man. There is unity in physical expression, in love and communication, and unity in emotion. Every emotion we feel is transmitted to *every* single cell of the body, and stored in the DNA. Everything we express and experience comes back to us on a cellular level. Each cell is affected by what we do or say. How incredible is that realization? This, again, ties us back to the power of our choices and actions, as we transcribe our own book of life everyday of our existence. When we can recognize this form of unity, we are motivated to make changes in our interactions with others, and the world around us.

The very world in which we live demonstrates unity. The interconnecting life cycles, or plants and animal life, teach us about unity. Seeds grow into plants, which then feed animals, and larger animals often feed on smaller animals, and upon cessation of their life, they return to the dust to provide more soil for plants to grow. The sun, and the moon and stars, work in concert to give constant light to the heavens, as they follow their rotation and orbit. The great waters are a collection of molecules that flow uniformly over the surface of the earth, and provide the lifeblood of the plants and vegetation. The clouds of the sky unify to produce precipitation, and return the evaporated waters from the earth.

Nothing is wasted in creation, everything has purpose and meaning, and everything is created to give and express in love. Can you imagine what the earth would be like if small animals were unwilling to sacrifice themselves to larger creatures of existence, or if seeds selfishly would not grow? What if the sun decided not to shine down on earth and bathe us with his light? How could we survive without the selfless acts of the creations on this earth? Yet, we are prone to selfishness and greed of our own making. Many of us desire to consume and compete, rather than to give and create. It is part of our existence that we must learn to overcome, if we are to completely heal our souls.

Often, as we venture into nature, we see this unity— we feel it even subconsciously, and it helps to alter our *own* natures. Being among the true patterns of creation of the universe, helps us tie ourselves into that very fabric, and ponder the deeper meanings of our life. This is often why the great outdoors can be one of the most refreshing and recommended prescriptions for our health. It is one of the most sacred places to feel unity.

Indeed, if you ever find yourself without supplements you've utilized to heal, I encourage you to try this exercise. Standing on

Mother Earth, close your eyes, and ask for renewal and rejuvenation from her. Imagine yourself as a tree, and let the roots from your feet branch down into the soil. Then imagine the minerals, vitamins, and other components that your body needs, come through the ground into your "roots," and disperse throughout the rest of your body. Indeed, when you have no access through physical means, according to your faith, you can access them metaphysically through the Spirit.

Additionally, when pure and clean water resources are scarce, you may ask for your water to be cleansed and purified. Specifically, ask that it become living water, which will further hydrate, rejuvenate, and cleanse your cells and body, allowing more light and love into your being. There is literally living water, and it is joyous, refreshing, and thirst quenching— symbolic of Jesus Christ.

An additional realization often comes when we are among the flora and fauna of this world. We recognize the peace from the busy tenets of life, and the freedom of expression. We are not inhibited from expressing our true selves in nature, because there is no one to judge us. In the peaceful silence, we revere the calm and quiet that is so essential to our well-being. Such an environment allows deep contemplation— and reverence for the beauty around us, and the connection that we are to creation.

We are meant to be the bridge between the physical and spiritual components of life, to bring them together as one. We do so by connecting physically and spiritually with our surroundings, and our fellow men. Often, we may deny this existence as one of unity, and try to experience life on our own. We try to handle everything by ourselves, and take on more and more projects to eliminate the need for social interaction.

We may have been deceived or injured by someone, and therefore, feel we can trust no one. Yet, we cannot deny that we are connected. As such, we are like a sea of emotion and experience that ripple, like the waves to the shore. We can feel the intentions of another, or their turmoil or worry. It connects us to humanity and wholeness, and can even be the cause of our physical distress! When we allow the emotions of others to affect our personal health, we are in disunion.

To promote unity, is to love those that are struggling or injured, or who have injured us. When we are able to fully forgive and love our fellow man, they can feel that love, and are inspired to change. It may not be an overnight manifestation, but it will happen. Using force to control or condemn another, will bring no joy or peace, and we will merely experience more of the same.

When we create our lives in love, there is no judgment of those around us. We can accept them for where they are in life, and recognize they are experiencing their own progression. As such, we can more readily foster their growth by recognizing their talents and abilities, and see their potential within. They, in turn, can shift into gratitude and service towards others. This positive ripple effect becomes a synergistic governance of complete equality and exchange, wherein, one is not above the other, but equal parts of the greater whole.

As we experience this unity among our fellows, it actually strengthens the unity of our soul! Literally, we heal on a physical and emotional level when we promote unity in our communities and nations. Our spiritual DNA, collectively, is altered, and more light is incorporated into the double helix.

When we experience fatigue, or are feeling down or unable to sleep— it is often because of disunion between the body and spirit. There may be physical causes, like adrenal dysfunction, or liver toxicity and pathogens, but some causes may be spiritual as well. We may be allowing another's emotions to weigh on us, and are taking it in like toxic fumes. We may be allowing another's judgment of us to alter our perception of our own worth as a divine being. We may be allowing pressure from others, guilt, distraction, or feelings of separation from God, to creep into our soul. We allow these thoughts to stifle our peace.

When these situations occur, it is a reflection that you are not viewing yourself as an equal to others, and are struggling with an inability to fully love yourself and others. As we are all equal, we are neither better, nor less than, another. We are one and the same. If we judge another, we are judging ourselves. If we completely forgive another, we are forgiving ourselves. If we have true compassion and charity towards another, we will do likewise for ourselves.

Exchanging emotions brings on a new dimension and meaning when viewed from this perspective. We all have heard the phrase, "what you reap, you sow," and this is a foundational truth! Yet, love is the ultimate expression of the universe, and if you want to absolve any and all negative emotions, you must call upon love in everything you do and are. Love is the way to disregard the judgment of another, or the negativity projected from them. When we can love ourselves deeply, as a child of God, we can transmit that love to others and forgo self-sabotage and criticism. Charity, the pure love of Christ, *never* fails.

Charity never faileth; but whether there be prophecies,
they shall fail; whether there be tongues, they shall cease;
whether there be knowledge, it shall vanish away.
1 Corinthians 13:8

Charity infuses our DNA with so much light, it can change gene expression entirely. Old genes, or "chapters" of negativity we inherited from our ancestry, can be altered and silenced with this love. If we live in love towards self and others everyday, there would be no place for illness to dwell! We would be full of so much light, there would be no darkness or disease. If you have been injured by another, validate your emotions are real, then work to release them, and give them to Christ. Forgo retention of that negativity, as it will not serve you to design your life in joy, but rather negatively impact gene expression.

So much of disunion resides in our desire for control. We are conditioned to want to control and command the elements of our life, to have predictability in all things. However, control will only project us so far in this life, and is of limited use for our growth. Indeed, it may promote an idea that your life is safe— but the reality is that you are limiting your ability to access greater power to create.

When we open up ourselves to the endless expanse of the universe, we are granted curiosity, innovation, and creativity. When we allow ourselves to be boxed in by limited ideas and progression, we are turning to the logic of our mind. We allow our logic to become the master of our universe, and it stifles creativity and expression. We were given dominion over the earth— we were meant to govern our creations. To govern does *not* mean to control— it means to behold, to witness, and to support.

As a healthcare provider, I recognize the limitations of control in medicine. I was taught in very black and white terms, regarding treatment options for illness. If you fit a check-box of symptoms, you were given a diagnosis, and prescribed the appropriate medication. Yet, if I had continued to ascribe to this ideology, I would not have been able to seek out additional insights to help patients. I would have remained stuck in a slow moving vehicle, based on evidence-based practices which are limited by physical extrapolation.

These evidence-based practices are derived from research of delineation and predictability, instead of innovation and creativity. Thus, I was limiting my abilities to help patients by only thinking inside the box. When I opened up to new possibilities, and sought instruction from Heavenly Father, my understanding was expanded into the unknown! Knowledge is limitless when we seek it out from the higher realms, but will be constricting if we only allow man's insight.

Terrenal instruction is helpful to explain patterns of creation— but it holds limitation, as we cannot physically see the end from the beginning. Taking the application to higher thought is essential to greater understanding and knowing. The more we do this, the more we can see and understand the greater aspect of unity within us, and each other. We become empowered, instead of limited, by temporal understanding, and can be a force for greater good on the earth.

Unity of the body and spirit, with God, man, and the universe, promotes powerful healing and miraculous insight! It is the perfect alignment to healing.

When we look at the pattern of the double helix, we see that it is in perfect unity. Apart from the time in which it is temporarily separated for transcription, it is bound together, coiled up, and protected, in the nuclear envelope. Not one amino acid base is left out; every single portion of the strand is included and cared for.

Symbolically, this represents us— each of us is cared for, protected, and watched over by God. We are not alone or forgotten, but indeed, are part of a greater whole, and we *are* connected to one another in a deep and abiding way, whether we recognize it or not. The sooner we understand this, and work towards greater unity, the stronger the bonds will be.

Like the double helix, our books of life can become seamlessly connected, and collectively cared for, by each of us. We can help one another return to the heavenly courts above, and be strengthened and renewed in the process. We obtain greater health and healing this way. When I was thinking about others in service, despite my illness, I was amazed to find that my symptoms were minimized during those times. I recognize now, that service and love bring a distinct change in our spiritual DNA that improves immune system health, and enhances our capability to fight the darkness of disease. The stronger our bonds of unity, the more protected and strengthened we will be, when disasters or disease occur in our lives.

Chapter **10**

Completion

To understand completion (or the end) we must first go to the beginning. I have always loved contemplating the atom and its resonance. The meaning of a smaller part, contributing to a greater whole, is awe inspiring and wondrous. I have always felt that there were even smaller units beyond the atom though, units that were so small, as to be invisible from man's capability to see it. When I learned about spiritual matter, this made perfect sense.

Spiritual matter is the finest unit of living matter that exists in the universe. It can be connected to physical matter, and form the earth, atmosphere, vegetation, animals, and humans. Spiritual and physical matter have always existed. This is where our divine origin took place, and whereupon we can build and create further. As intelligences, we followed likewise— starting out as spiritual matter, growing to receive a spirit body, and then receiving a physical body, in the flesh, from God. We derived from these particles of spiritual matter!

As these particles are endless, so are we. Even upon cessation of our lives on this earth, we begin living anew elsewhere. Everything we have learned and experienced will carry with us into the next realm. We leave a personal mark, or "name," on our creations, and they become remembered in our spiritual DNA.

On a particular scale, we have been discussing the spiritual

DNA, the ladder of life, with all of its chapters and books. On an even smaller scale, the DNA is comprised of elements, then atoms, and then these particles of spiritual elements. Factually then, the whole essence of humanity (us) is woven together in the DNA. We are connected to each other through this concept, and it has a real and predictive value of love. The love of Christ and His sacrifice made it possible to be unified forever in this way. This is what permits us to feel as others feel, and see as they see, to have empathy towards them, and their circumstance.

Our DNA is connected to the genes of deity, and as such, we have the potential to become like our Heavenly Father (God) in *every* way. It is granted unto us to have agency, the power to choose. We have the power to open or close, genes or "chapters" of our book, dependent upon how we choose to feel, think, and act. Love is the highest power and frequency of all, and through it (via sincere repentance and obedience), our spiritual DNA can be shifted and turned towards God.

We each knew what we came here to do prior to this mortal experience, and we were excited to come and prove ourselves. We knew that there would be separation, sadness, pain, and suffering— but also great joy, excitement, pleasure, and peace. We knew that in the end, we could return home where our book of life would be reviewed. To those who did their best to follow Christ, and keep His commandments— they are promised eternal happiness, and further progression. They will have inexpressible joy and gratitude to be with loved ones. Christ's suffering on their behalf, will satisfy the demands of justice, and they will be allowed to enter His presence. To those who chose not to follow Him and accept His sacrifice, they are turned over to the fullness of justice, and will be cut off from God's presence.

"What, do ye suppose that mercy can rob justice? I say unto you nay, not one whit. If so, God would cease to be God."
Alma 42:25

God follows through on His every word, and He must execute justice for those who did not follow His laws. Some believe they can do whatever they want to in this life, and there will be no consequence. This is a grossly mistaken belief, and our current mortal experience negates this ideology. We cannot believe that we won't be held accountable for choosing to do things contrary to God's word, just as we cannot escape a speeding ticket by breaking terrenal laws.

To demean, depress, or destroy others, will truly bring condemnation on those who choose to behave thus. To those who have darkened their souls, to the extent they feel no remorse to repent— your spiritual DNA will testify against you in the end. You will be your own judge, as all your wicked works are written on your very sinews.

To such individuals— I encourage you to make the decision *now* to change. It is far easier to make restitution in this life. Otherwise, there is a place of burning, anguish, and self-deprecation, that will be endless for you in the eternity to come. Thus will be your state of "completion," if you do not choose to repent now.

"The Son of man shall send forth his angels, and they shall gather out of his kingdom all things that offend, and them which do iniquity; And shall cast them into a furnace of fire: there shall be wailing and gnashing of teeth. Then shall the righteous shine forth as the sun in the kingdom of their Father. Who hath ears to hear, let him hear."
Matthew 13: 41-43

Completion can have many meanings. It can identify a time of cessation, wherein all things are finished. When we view it in this light, we understand that there have been many phases of completion in this world. The creation of the earth was finished millennia ago. We all have been granted mortal completion by receiving a body, and the Atonement of Jesus Christ, has been accomplished. Many of our beloved family and friends have already completed their mortal lives, and await us on the other side.

Everyday, we take one step further to the completion of our work here on the earth. It is up to us to determine how that completion will occur. We have the opportunity to choose how to live our life, and what to include in its creation. We are creating and completing something everyday of mortality— is not that a thrilling thought? It is wonderful to reflect on all you've created and completed in your lifetime.

We are beings of creation, indeed— it is part of our DNA. Our thoughts promote our actions, which then create experiences! All too often, we think of creating *only* as being something visible and tactile that can be witnessed from start to finish. Yet, there are many ways we create and complete without raw materials. Memories, relationships, and emotions, are all creations without physical properties! These are accomplishments that we rarely give any notice to, but they are the essence of our lives.

As a Creator, are you also a Completer? The author *and* finisher of our faith empowered us to follow through on the promises that we made prior to this life. When we are going through a trial of health, we tend to make that the only focus of our life. It is so difficult to find the balance, wherein we are doing all we can to heal, while not forgetting the *purpose* of our life! Chronic illness often gives us tunnel vision, yet it can be a blessed reminder of who we are, and what we are here to do.

Despite the difficulty of the way, we can recognize that we are still in a process of creating and calling into our purview what we need to learn, even while we are ill. We can realize completion *every* day, as we understand something new on our healing journey. It may be learning how to eat healthier, or understanding the amazing properties of plants. It could be improving your communication with God, or more fully recognizing your divine potential and power. It could include learning to be optimistic in the face of opposition, looking outside ourselves to serve— despite our personal plights, and making memories of laughter, despite the pain.

Indeed, we can create *and* complete something everyday. It is important to celebrate the little victories of completion we experience on our healing journey. It may be getting a shower in that day, or sending a heartfelt message to another. It may even be praying a little more sincerely, waiting a little more patiently, and giving a little more graciously. It also can be improvement of physical symptoms over a period of time. Every little positive observance should be recorded and appreciated, and can give us motivation on harder days.

When we feel poorly, we often look forward to rapid recovery. It, by nature, is the focus or goal of intent. We view illness as a process we merely must endure and "deal" with, until we magically regain our strength. To be chronically ill is abhorred, and even feared. As a society, we've even begun to blame others for their chronic ailments. Because of this negative connotation, many forgo finding the deeper, divine principles by which they can be made whole.

Seeking out a quick fix, they may find temporary improvement, but longer-term sequela inevitably ensues. If we could turn the paradigm around, it would promote powerful healing. If we viewed any illness as an invitation to support and sustain the body's healing processes, while positively engaging the spirit and mind, we would see remarkable results. We could understand that it is an opportunity for growth in faith, endurance, and dedication, unlike any other. We could recognize that some of the strongest souls are given challenges with chronic illness, and we could appreciate their wisdom and insight.

Collectively, we could support one another to heal in a more communal way. Faith would grow, stronger discernment would develop, and more miracles would manifest. We would see greater completion of healing, in a shorter period of time, based on these principles.

Another source of completion, is when the spiritual DNA (our life experience) is fully transcribed, and the time of reckoning to God has arrived. Each of us has our time here on earth fixed, and it is varied for every individual. God knows when we will be called home to report our completions of creation. We do not know His timing, although some may have personal promptings, prior to their decease. Regardless, it is important to note that we need to live our life in the *present*.

Now is the day to do our best and learn what we can. If we focus too far in the future, we forgo creating the experiences of today. If we are dwelling in the past, we are preventing forward progression. Life is not easy, it was never meant to be. It is a thrilling roller-coaster ride of ups and downs, incredible insights, and difficult trials. No one will have a simple, easy existence, without any difficulty— otherwise, mortality would be worthless.

There will be physical, emotional, and spiritual suffering, as each of us face different challenges. Some face hidden addictions and deceptions, while others have a more visible trial. Yet, despite all of this, we are learning and growing in experience. We will have easier days and harder days, but how we perceive them is important. If we recognize we have learned and progressed already over multiple millennia, to become what we are now, it helps us recognize that this earth life is extremely short in duration! It helps us to remember the end result of completion, and we can strive to learn through each challenge, as we seek guidance from above.

The most beautiful thing is how *everything* is orchestrated for each individual— every experience and challenge is tailored specifically to you, to your interests and abilities, and to what you wanted to learn to progress. There are moments in your life where you can reflect back and recognize how much you have grown; what you have learned and overcome— it is a beautiful tapestry and testimony of your life. Woven on the loom of discernment, it will be yours to keep forever.

This prospect of completion may be disconcerting for some. They may view it as a looming final in their last college math class, on which hinges their graduation and degree. But if we think of it as thus, we will forget all the amazing classes we've taken, and the great friends we've encountered along the way. We won't recall the helpful professors who gave us guidance, and how they opened our views to something new. We will forgo remembrance of the late night cramming and caffeine fixes that got us through to graduation. We may even forget all the support and love we received from family members, as we completed our work.

To those who have graduated from any program or school, you can recognize that the rewarding feeling that comes with graduation does *not* come from the ceremony itself. It comes from what *you did* to get there. The sacrifices and struggles, the blood, sweat, and tears that you gave towards its accomplishment. Thus it is with our life. If we choose to find joy in the journey, we will not only learn greater lessons, and transcribe our spiritual DNA in greater light and knowledge, but we will have a greater impact on those around us. This life is purposeful, it is useful— and it is difficult. But it is also exciting, fun, and inspiring too, as we pause to take in the view from the climb.

Miracles of complete healing by Christ are depicted in scripture. These personal miracles are still occurring today, despite them not being as publicly known. I testify these miracles do, and will, exist, and will increase in frequency— as we obtain the faith sufficient to be healed. Miracles such as these occur through the power of God, and bring complete resolution to one's illness. As noted in scripture, the soul can obey the command to be made whole.

When you receive the love and light of God, in such abundance that your body is so full of light, any and all darkness can be obliterated from the body. This is the highest state of healing, and is done by your spirit, in conjunction with the power of God. This is more powerful, than any scientific modality on the planet, to heal a person. This supersedes medical innovations and new prescriptions. This even amasses the power of fruits, vegetables, and herbs in their power and ability to help us heal.

This is a Celestial level of healing that transcends any current knowledge on the planet. This level of healing requires personal responsibility, and a willingness to work to develop the stature of faith necessary to take the leap. It is a beautiful process, wherein we develop complete and total trust in God, and learn to go directly to the source of all truth in everything we do. It is an opportunity to sift through the philosophies and ideas of men, and find God's truth in all things, as we walk His path to healing.

It is a modality that can heal spiritual, emotional, and physical ailments, simultaneously and completely. It is a life changing process, and miraculous to behold. God desires all of His children, who suffer from any pain or distress, to observe and obtain this type of healing. It is an opportunity extended towards all, and is possible to obtain, if one is not appointed unto death. However, He will always meet His children where they are at, and offer support at every level. From personal experience, I am grateful for every modality, and utilized each one through my journey to heal. But I am infinitely grateful to have experienced Celestial healing. He made up for what I could *not* do to heal myself. It has changed my life entirely, and I will never forget the miracle it is.

We are living in an exciting, and yet tempestuous time. The earth is being prepared for the return of our Savior, and is nearing her completion. There will be great trials and tribulations for all of us, and yet it will be incredibly joyous as well. We can work towards our completion, as we walk hand in hand with the finisher of our faith. He is our Creator *and* Completer, and we can come to Him for strength, succor, and stamina. We can find resiliency and repose in His arms. I promise you as you adhere to the correct principles to truly heal *now*, you will reap greater benefits— now *and* in the future. In time, you may be prompted to call upon God with unshakeable faith for deliverance— and He will heal you.

Epilogue

I have felt impressed to include some examples of healing by faith in scripture. The purpose of this is to illustrate variances among healing modalities and experiences, while also identifying the common thread of faith among those who were healed. It is my hope you may gain insight into your own healing journey through these historical accounts.

First, let us consider the "woman with the issue of blood," in Luke 8:43-48. This woman had dealt with heavy bleeding for over twelve years and had spent *everything* she had on physicians. She had likely gone to multiple providers, searching for answers, trying multiple modalities, changing her diet, taking herbs, and following the counsel given to her. Yet none of these things worked, and her condition actually worsened. (Mark 5:25-26) However, she did not give up hope and actually grew in faith through this process. She still believed that she could heal, and she continued to search. Hearing of Jesus, she purposely sought Him out, *knowing* He could heal her. She had done everything she could do— and by touching His garment, she was made whole. This can apply to us as well— we may be required to do everything we can do, seek out all modalities, try a variety of things and not give up on our faith. Our journey to heal may not be immediate, but more prolonged. Yet, we can grow in patience, long-suffering, service, and temperance and obtain greater faith until *we* are made whole.

Next, we look to Namaan the leper (Kings 5:1-14). He was a

powerful man and many revered him, yet he was struck with leprosy. Hearing of a prophet in Israel who could heal him, he besought his King to inquire on his behalf. Upon receipt of the King's request, Elisha invited Namaan to come and see him. He obeyed, and came with all his horses and his chariot (it must have been quite the spectacle); but he must have been surprised when he was not met by Elisha himself. Instead, Elisha sent a servant to him, and instructed him that he should bathe in the River Jordan seven times. He was promised that if he did so, he would be made whole. Initially, Namaan was angry, and would not do as he was asked. He expected a great miracle to occur, as the prophet called upon the powers of heaven to heal him instantly. Because of his pride, he was about to let an incredible opportunity to demonstrate his faith go to waste. Yet, he hearkened to his servants who counseled him to obey. Upon the seventh time washing in the river, he was completely healed and praised God.

This story can illustrate how pride can deter a person from pursuing the correct path to healing. All too often, we pursue extensive testing, expensive treatments, and the most cutting edge procedures to help us heal. We want immediate results. Fads and trends take hold and we may want to follow along. However, it may be that healing occurs by small and simple means, daily consistency with sound dietary and exercise regimes, and obedience to God's counsel to us. Sometimes we may be instructed to do something that sounds too simple to us, but as we obey we are blessed.

Lastly, I wish to discuss the man born blind (John 9:1-7). During his earthly ministry, Jesus saw a man who was blind from birth. His disciples asked him who had sinned- the man, or his parents, to bring such a plight upon him. Jesus replied that neither had sinned, but it was orchestrated so that the "works of God should be made manifest in him" (John 9:3). Then, Jesus spat in the dirt and made mud, which he then applied to the blind man's eyes. Afterward, he instructed the man to go and wash in the waters of Siloam. The man obeyed, and received a restoration of his sight.

There is a great deal of meaning to this encounter. First, we learn that illness is not necessarily a result of sin. We should never assume that an ill person is sick because they brought it on themselves, or think that they aren't trying hard enough, or that it is "all in their head" because they look fine on the outside. We can realize that illness is part of life, and it is an opportunity for us to learn how to access the powers of heaven to heal, that the works of God may be manifest in *us*. When considering this event, we may think that the manifestation of God's work, in this situation, was the miracle of restoring physical sight.

However, have you paused to consider that it could also include a restoration of the man's spiritual sight, of being redeemed from spiritual darkness and receiving greater light and knowledge? Thus, "manifesting the works of God" can include our transformation to demonstrate greater faith, to receive greater knowledge, to have deeper compassion and gratitude, and to serve with greater purpose throughout our trial of illness- however long it may last. The *miracle* of such personal transformation is even greater when accompanied by personal sorrow, pain and suffering. Remember this- *you* are already a miracle, by choosing to serve and lift those around you, despite your illness.

Another important point to ponder is that the blind man could do nothing of his own volition to heal. He was blind from birth; there was no remedy that could physically be incorporated to reverse the problem. Even so, the Lord required him to *act* in faith. It was a tender mercy for the Lord to recognize that perhaps the man had dealt with his malady for so long, that he had not faith *yet* sufficient to be healed. However, by applying the clay spittle and instructing him to wash in Siloam, he was giving the man an opportunity to increase his faith, by following His words. Do we recognize that our illness may be an invitation to demonstrate our willingness to follow God's counsel, in order to gain the faith to be healed? Do we follow the spirit's guidance even if it doesn't make sense? When the path to healing is hard, and the skies seem to darken- do we hold on to hope, or choose to throw in the towel? I find it interesting that in so many accounts of healing in scripture, the individual acted *immediately* and followed Christ's counsel. They did not delay, or disbelieve, but did as they were told.

It has caused me to wonder if Christ healed everyone He encountered, or if there was a pattern and purpose to these healing blessings. I personally feel that He healed those who had faith in *Him* and His power to heal, who wanted so badly to believe in Him, they would sacrifice anything to receive such a miracle. To those whose faith was not sufficient, or whose faith wavered— He could not heal.

It is my hope that you have gained greater insight and inspiration that will allow you to ponder, pray, and act on the counsel you receive from Heaven. You are worth *everything* to God, and He and His angels are watching, and waiting to assist you. I know you can heal— and now you do too. I end this with my testimony that I know that God lives, and I know Jesus is the Christ! He is real, resurrected, and loves you personally. I promise you, that as you seek to find Him, He will guide you along your path to return home— healed and whole. There is no wound so deep, no pain so great, no suffering so sore that He *cannot* heal. May we one day meet before our Maker and rejoice in His goodness and glory. In the sacred name of Jesus Christ, Amen.

Appendix of Spiritual Genes (not exhaustive)

Genes of Adam
Genes of Eve
Genes of faith (in God, self, Christ, others)
Genes of fortitude
Genes of gratitude
Genes of resiliency
Genes of peace
Genes of presence
Genes of procreation
Genes of mindfulness
Genes of despair
Genes of compassion
Genes of hope
Genes of love (for self, God, Christ)
Genes of trust- in self, others, God
Genes of fear (silence)
Genes of affirmation
Genes of light
Genes of dissention (silence)
Genes of doubt (silence)
Genes of belief
Genes of direction

Genes of deliverance
Genes of obedience
Genes of charity (for self, others, God)
Genes of Remembrance
Genes of laughter
Genes of humor
Genes of desire to (serve, persist, etc)
Genes of Unity

Bibliography

Pontius, John. *Following the Light of Christ Into His Presence.* Springville: Cedar Fort Incorporated, 2014. Print

William, Anthony. *The Medical Medium: Secrets to Chronic and Mystery Illness and How to Finally Heal.* Carlsbad: Hay House Incorporated, 2015. Print